...emove a spinal tumour left him almost ...pain. His career as a university teacher ended, his p...e...s...itions were thwarted and his active social life was completely wiped out. These events left him in a state of despair and helplessness, as he struggled to pick up the pieces, heal the resulting emotional scars, restore hope and regain a satisfactory quality of life. Over the past 30 years, Neville has not only helped himself but has worked as a therapist and author to help others to find ways to rebuild their lives. He believes that people have power to help themselves and others to cope with adversity. His books, *Coping Successfully with Pain, Cancer – a Family Affair, The Chronic Pain Diet Book* and *The Pain Management Handbook* (all published by Sheldon Press), continue to act as a source of inspiration. Neville has broadcast on local and national radio and television on the subject of pain management, and has acted as a consultant to a number of television documentary makers. He is patron to two national pain charities. A graduate of the University of Liverpool, he returned there to teach after a career in social work with children and families. He is qualified as a psychotherapist and hypnotherapist. Neville is married to Eve, and much of the couple's time and energy is spent with their children, grandchildren and thirteen great-grandchildren.

A full list of titles is availa[ble]
36 Causton Street, London SW1[P]
www.sheldonpress.co[.uk]

Overcoming Common Problems

Coping Successfully with Chronic Illness
Your healing plan

NEVILLE SHONE

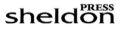

First published in Great Britain in 2013

Sheldon Press
36 Causton Street
London SW1P 4ST
www.sheldonpress.co.uk

British Library Cataloguing-in-Publication Data
A catalogue record for this book is available from the British Library

ISBN 978–1–84709–228–1
eBook ISBN 978–1–84709–229–8

Typeset by Caroline Waldron, Wirral, Cheshire
First printed in Great Britain by Ashford Colour Press
Subsequently digitally printed in Great Britain

Produced on paper from sustainable forests

*This book is dedicated to my grandchildren and
great-grandchildren, in the hope that they will read it
to discover more about their family history,
and that they will enjoy a life full of health and happiness*

A flawed diamond is more valuable than a perfect brick.
(Anon.)

Contents

Acknowledgements

I wish to acknowledge the help I have received over the years from the many people who have contributed to my own quest for healing. Their contribution has given me the knowledge, energy and will to pass on all that I learned from them. In particular, thanks are due to Dr Christopher Wells, former Director of the Pain Management Programme at Walton Hospital, Liverpool; the late Helen Yaffe who did so much to rekindle my failing spirits and show me the way forward; David Falconer, Director, Pain Association Scotland, for his encouragement and friendship over many years; and Rosanne Falconer for her generous contribution to this book.

Thanks are also due to Marcello Lowther, practitioner of Advanced Remedial Massage, Sports and Manipulative Therapy, for his continuing contribution to my well-being and comfort and his valuable advice, and to Sarah Wrigley for sharing her experience of coping with MS and life in general.

My thanks also go to those others whose experiences are included in this book. Their names and certain details have been changed in order to protect their privacy. All of them have helped in their own way to further my own knowledge about the healing process.

Once again I would like to thank Joanna Moriarty, Editorial Director, and Fiona Marshall, Commissioning Editor, Sheldon Press. Fiona has provided invaluable help and encouragement in working out a focus for this book.

I wish to thank Diet Freedom Ltd for allowing me to use their recipe for Avocado Chocolate Mousse with Strawberries (see page 89).

Author's note to the reader

If you have any kind of medical problem you must consult your doctor.

The material in this book is to help you to maximize your own health and well-being. It is not intended to replace any advice given by your own medical practitioner. The author can accept no responsibility for actions you undertake as a result of reading this book.

Introduction

I was sitting alone in an old Victorian hospital ward. It had until recently been used as a sewing room by the housekeeping staff. It seemed to be a curious setting for the first pain management course in the UK and Europe, staffed by a team of doctors, psychologists, occupational and physical therapists as well as teachers of dance and yoga. This highly skilled and strongly motivated team had volunteered to work with chronic pain patients who had been 'written off' when standard medicine had no more to offer in way of treatment.

The room was shabby and sparsely furnished with a few old wooden and plastic chairs scrounged from various parts of the hospital. There were two reasonably comfortable, if battered, armchairs. The floor was covered in brown cracked linoleum from a bygone age. In one corner was a table containing about a dozen coffee mugs, an electric kettle, a tin of instant coffee, a box of teabags, a carton of milk, a bag of sugar and a few spoons. Behind a curtain on the opposite side of the room was an examination table. It was the middle of winter, cloudy and wet outside, and because no lights were on it was extremely dismal inside as well. In this large depressing room with its high ceiling I felt very insignificant, helpless and hopeless.

I was waiting for the arrival of 'Helen the Healer', one of the team of therapists, and I had no idea what to expect. I was beginning the second week of my pain management course and the only feedback I had from the other seven patients who were my companions on the course, and were by now on their third and final week, was that they all felt better as a result of seeing her. They hinted at the release of strong emotions and feelings of extreme heat in various parts of their body.

I had been brought up to think that all healing came from the medical profession, espousing the latest in scientific medicine, drugs and surgical procedures. However, my faith in their abilities had been badly shaken by my own experience of long waiting lists, delays in diagnosis, lost notes, drugs to which I was allergic and an operation which left me with severe chronic pain, walking difficulties and extreme discomfort when standing or sitting. At this point I had little faith in anyone to improve my condition.

All I knew about healing outside the medical profession came from my studies of anthropology, highlighting the work of witch doctors and shamans, and modern depictions of preachers from the Bible Belt of America dramatically driving out demons from the possessed. Understandably, I was extremely apprehensive about giving myself over to 'witchcraft' but at the same time I was so desperate to achieve some relief from my pain that I was prepared to listen to anyone who might be able to help me.

Even after such a short time on the pain management course I knew that something was happening to me that indicated some improvement. What it was I was not sure at this stage, because my pain and mobility were still much the same. I had had a week learning how to breathe properly and how to relax deeply, and had followed a daily programme of progressive exercise. I tried to analyse the cause of this change. It was something I had not experienced before. Our group of eight was led through a series of guided discussions and activities and everyone was given space and time to express their views, their feelings and their hopes for the immediate and long-term future. Was it the group itself that was bringing about a change in my feelings? Was it the flow of endorphins coming from the unaccustomed exercise and relaxation sessions? My professional background in working with children and families, teaching social work and probation officer students about groups and leading therapeutic groups told me that the group is a very powerful instrument in bringing about change for the better. However, I was not there just to feel better. I *needed* to have less pain and I *needed* to be more mobile. When was this going to happen?

I learned from those running the course, and the other attendees, that if we were going to progress we were going to have to work very hard at physical conditioning. It involved not only training muscles that had been unused for more than five years and straightening a body that had become twisted but also re-learning the fundamentals of walking and sitting, while at the same time finding ways to change many aspects of our behaviour, our habits and our ways of relating to people. This was only the beginning, where we learned the necessary skills to use as a foundation we could build on when the course finished in four weeks. Do-it-yourself was the order of the day!

Support lasted as long as the group was together, but once you graduated you were on your own. I saw this as the crisis point – learn the skills and survive, or go under! I got the message that the medical profession generally still had very little to offer in treating chronic pain. Would I fare any better with this new approach to treatment? At this stage it was hard to believe that the small gains

I had made in the first two weeks of the course would continue – and for how long?

My thoughts were interrupted by the door opening. In walked a very ordinary-looking woman, perhaps mid-50s, greying, but with a bright smile which lit up the dim room. Introductions over, we sat down and Helen told me she had missed the chance to meet me the first week I was on the course. This was because she had been away 'recharging her batteries'. She explained that working intensively with people could be very exhausting, and I knew this well from my own work experience with students and families suffering breakdown. We had an immediate point of contact. She went on to say her work with me had nothing to do with my religious experience or faith or the intervention of some outside force, but she was there to focus my own energy so that I could use it to strengthen my own ability to heal myself. She asserted that the only sure healing came from within, but that life experience and illness can so easily overwhelm the ability we all have to mend damage to the mind and body. I could relate to this. It made sense to me, as for the last few years my illness had taken such a grip on me that I had no time or energy left for other things.

Helen then invited me to choose whether to lie on the examination couch, to stand up or to sit down, whichever was more comfortable for me. Standing was out of the question and I felt too vulnerable to lie on a couch (too much like the Hollywood version of visiting a psychiatrist). I chose to sit on one of the plastic chairs, not normally a comfortable experience for me.

Helen stood behind me and explained that she would take a little time to scan my body with her hands, but no contact would be made. I could not see how this would help my pain. I had expected some form of 'the laying on of hands' but this did not happen. Instead, she raised her hands, one to the front and one to the back of my head just about three inches away. As she did so she said, 'You *know* what to do,' and began to scan slowly down my torso. I didn't understand her remark – or so I thought. The only thing I could think she meant was that I should close my eyes and breathe slowly into my diaphragm as I had been taught in the relaxation classes. As she scanned, I was very aware of the position of her hands through a sensation of warmth. (You can experience this for yourself by holding the palms of your hands about three inches apart and closing your eyes. This is an excellent way to relax, especially if you slow down your breathing at the same time.) The feeling of warmth and relaxation was all I could

feel, until she reached my midriff area. Nothing had prepared me
for what happened next.

I experienced an enormous knot of tension in my chest that
completely interrupted my ability to breathe smoothly. I felt
myself gasping for breath, sweating, and I was overtaken by an
upsurge of emotion expressed in tears. I gasped out, 'I don't know
where that came from.' I was possessed by these strong feelings
for some time and I began to talk about all the things that I had
bottled up over a number of years: my feelings of letting down the
family; my anger at the loss of my job, my income, my status, my
hobbies; my confusion and fear for my future and my sanity.

We talked about these things for what seemed like an age. It was
the first time I had talked about my feelings and anxieties, and I
realized I had been spending so much time and energy putting on
a brave face to convince those around me that I was coping. This
was the first time I had admitted to anyone that I was not coping
– that I was terrified and helpless and saw the future as being completely black. Helen picked up on this. She said that she liked to
work with colours and asked me to see if I could bring about any
change mentally by altering the black into something brighter.
As I focused my mind I noticed my breathing slowing down and
becoming much deeper. I began to sweat profusely, and it seemed
an age before I experienced flashes of colour at the edges of the
blackness. Flashes of purple . . . changing to blue . . . which eventually and after much concentration and mental effort . . . began
to push away much of the blackness. With encouragement from
Helen I continued and finally was able to fill the black space with
whiteness. At this point I felt an overwhelming sense of euphoria
– a wonderful feeling of achievement – and I felt a flow of energy
begin to flood through my body, bringing with it exhilaration and
joy, feelings I had forgotten and never expected to regain. I was
soaking with sweat and felt completely exhausted.

These strong, positive feelings stayed with me throughout the
following week when I was able to feel more involved with my
family and put more energy into the pain management course. I
looked forward to my next session with Helen.

I cannot recall in absolute detail everything that happened in
the following session but I do remember that it was just as intense
and just as exhilarating. It ended with me walking triumphantly
from one end of the room to the other without the aid of sticks
and without stooping or limping. And what followed was even
more unexpected. Helen showed me into the corridor and urged

me to climb the grand Victorian staircase to the next floor. I started hesitantly, thinking Helen was being too ambitious and that there would be tears before bedtime. However, she had thrown down the gauntlet, I was desperate to succeed and I was not one to shirk a challenge. Deep down I trusted Helen enough to know she would not put me in danger. With each step my confidence grew, even though I could feel the strength draining from my legs. I was shaking from head to foot by the time I reached the landing but, for the first time in five years, I was fully mobile!

Looking back, I can only describe this as a truly healing experience, but not in the sense of being 'cured'. More than 30 years on I still have my spinal condition, I still have chronic pain, allergies and mobility problems, but what I experienced in those meetings with Helen was so intense and positive that it was really life-changing. For the first time I saw the possibility that I could move on, and this enabled me to break free from being dominated by my illness and to plan ahead without fear or anxiety.

Anyone who is chronically sick who reaches the stage where it is possible to think positively about the future with confidence is well on the way to being healed.

What was gloom is now bright; where there was once helplessness there is a feeling of control; where there was once despair there is hope. These new positive feelings did not come all at once, but over the following days and months I began to become less focused on my physical body and its defects. I began to pick up on family relationships, take more interest in things going on around me, set myself goals and feel confident enough to grasp opportunities. In spite of the fact that I still had reservations about my physical capacities I was delighted when I was asked to make a contribution to the pain management programme, using my skills in group therapy that I had practised as a family social worker and taught for many years as a university teacher. This was the start of a new career for me, as very soon I was able to retrain, over a period of three years, as a psychotherapist and hypnotherapist and run my own practice treating individual patients. I found my new skills invaluable in working with the endless procession of people with pain when they were referred to the increasingly popular and effective pain management programme.

I soon learned that many of the people seeking help, whether coming to me for individual attention or attending the pain management course, were suffering from a variety of chronic illnesses and were desperate to find some relief from their pain, anxiety, sleeplessness, stress and depression. As time went on I felt that the focus of my work was not so much towards treatment as towards education, enabling my 'students' to use and enhance their own inner resources, learning new coping skills and ways of thinking and behaving in order to bring about their own healing. The more students were able to embrace this new learning and incorporate it into their daily lives, the more it was possible to see real changes taking place as they were able to find ways of conquering some if not all of the troublesome symptoms of their illness. As I developed this educational approach more, I thought that it would be helpful to conduct such a course in the community away from all the usual connotations of hospital, white coats, disease, trauma, high tech equipment and emphasis on drugs. In my first book *Coping Successfully with Pain* (Sheldon, 2002) I have described how it was possible to work in this way.

Human beings are extremely complex, and in the case of chronic illness it is arrogant to think that it is sufficient to treat only the physical body. There is a complex interaction between the mind, thoughts, feelings, spirit and physiology of a person. Life experience can disrupt this process, giving rise to chronic illness. In this book I hope to throw some light on how this can happen and demonstrate how it is possible for you to learn how to work towards restoring ease within yourself so you can enjoy an enhanced quality of life. I hope you will discover, through following the plan I have devised, how to make good things happen throughout your life.

Chronic illness – a global problem, a personal challenge

A global problem

Chronic illness is a malady that persists for a long time. It is commonly accepted in the medical profession that any illness that lasts for over three months can be described as chronic. Many of us have experienced acute illnesses that, in spite of causing discomfort, inconvenience and anxiety, come and go quickly. Such illnesses are chest infections, stomach infections, colds and influenza. To put the subject of chronic illness in perspective I turned to the publications of the World Health Organization (WHO), which monitors health trends throughout the world and from time to time makes recommendations for the guidance of the countries that make up its membership. I must admit I was taken aback when I read the statistics about the extent and profound effects of chronic illness.

The WHO reported that in 2005 chronic conditions such as heart disease, diabetes, stroke, cancer and chronic respiratory diseases were by far the leading cause of mortality in the world, representing 60 per cent of all deaths. Of the 35 million who died from chronic disease in that year, half were under 70. The WHO describes this as an 'invisible epidemic, an underappreciated cause of poverty and a hindrance to the economic development of many countries'.

In a document entitled 'Facing the Facts: The impact of chronic disease in the United Kingdom', the WHO reports that chronic diseases are projected to account for 85 per cent of all deaths between 2005 and 2015, in numerical terms five million people. In the same period, although it is estimated that the overall percentage dying from chronic illness will fall by 0.8 per cent, deaths from some chronic illnesses will increase. The report draws attention specifically to diabetes where the estimated increase is said to be 25 per cent.

1

The WHO report also points out that being overweight and obese is a major cause of chronic disease. In the ten years from 2005 to 2015 the number of overweight and obese men in the population will increase from 76 per cent to 80 per cent, with the percentage for women projected to rise from 69 to 73 per cent.

In economic terms, in 2005 alone premature deaths from heart disease, stroke and diabetes lost the UK $2 billion in national income (the WHO uses the dollar as a common reference point in order to compare costs from one country to another). In the years 2005 to 2015 the loss to the UK economy is projected to increase to $33 billion as a result of premature deaths from heart disease, stroke and diabetes.

The WHO suggests that a healthy diet, regular physical activity and avoidance of tobacco products would make major inroads into the prevalence of these diseases and also cancer.

The WHO report refers only to the obviously life-threatening illnesses but there are many other chronic illnesses that need to be taken into account. These, in their turn, are known to have a major economic impact. Chronic pain alone affects more than eight and a half million people in the UK and costs the economy £18 billion in lost working days each year. The charity Arthritis Care carried out research in 2012 that predicts the number of people with osteoarthritis will double over the next few years, mainly as a result of obesity and the growing number of aged people in the community.

A personal challenge

Other conditions that fall under the definition of chronic illness and which may be making your life miserable or stressful and preventing you from living life to the full may include:

- one of the many forms of arthritis and joint problems
- osteoporosis
- spondylitis and spondylosis
- spinal stenosis
- fibromyalgia
- myalgic encephalopathy (ME), also known as chronic fatigue syndrome (CFS)
- multiple sclerosis (MS)
- neuralgia – for example trigeminal neuralgia, post-herpetic neuralgia (pain after shingles), post-operative adhesions and adhesions following injury

- cancer and cancer pain following treatment
- stress, anxiety and depression
- high blood pressure and chronic heart disease
- insomnia
- migraine
- digestive problems
- irritable bowel syndrome (IBS)
- dermatitis, eczema, psoriasis
- chest complaints and asthma and other chronic conditions.

While not always directly life-threatening, any of these conditions can take away our zest for life, sap our energy and virtually extinguish that inner flame that we call 'spirit'. Some people suggest that it is the weakening of the spirit that is the root cause of many illnesses; however, this is not the place to get into a chicken-or-egg debate as the main purpose of this book is to help you to heal, to strengthen your spirit and your body and to use your mind to help your personal transformation.

The weakening of the spirit can make it difficult to take action to help yourself overcome problems arising from the illness, and these can be legion. There may be unpleasant symptoms to deal with which get progressively worse in spite of medication or treatment, resulting in feelings of frustration, helplessness and hopelessness. You may see aspects of your life just melting away as it becomes more difficult to hold down a job or do everyday tasks about the home. Hobbies and social life and – even worse – relationships may fall victim to your illness and you may feel isolated and alone as you are unable to share your fears and worries with friends or loved ones. You may indulge in self-blame or feel unable to follow through a rigid programme of treatment.

Getting back to living an enjoyable life in spite of your illness presents a real challenge. You may find it easier to sit back and do nothing rather than face making changes that are an essential prelude to following a programme that will help you get better. You may believe you are beyond help or you may feel it is a sign of inadequacy or failure to seek help; you may not want to trouble your doctor – it might seem you are complaining that the treatment you are receiving is no good. After all, Doctor knows best! You may already have exhausted the treatment options provided by conventional medicine. You might feel that you are to blame for the inactivity resulting from your illness that has culminated in substantial weight gain, and be afraid to have someone sit in judgement over you. These and other barriers may prevent you from seeking the help you need or taking steps to help yourself – even if you knew what they were. Or you may take a different approach and react to your illness by seeking help from many sources, desperate to find a cure, putting yourself in the hands of anyone eager to take your money and ending up disappointed and maybe near to bankruptcy.

Be assured that most people find ways to cope – with or without help.

Most of us take time to adjust to a personal crisis, whatever it may be: bereavement, separation or divorce, loss of home or job, or the onset of an illness. These life events usually present a challenge we have not met before and our ability to cope is limited because we have not developed any coping skills or strategies to deal with them. Even if we have coping skills as a result of meeting similar challenges in the past we are unable to call on them immediately. All such events produce strong emotions that can temporarily overwhelm us and make us incapable of taking action. It seems that time is needed for the emotional shock to be absorbed, processed and made sense of before we are ready to move on and devise ways of handling the situation. Even then, several solutions may need to be tried before we feel we have made a satisfactory adjustment. Sometimes, as we shall see in Chapter 5, these emotional events can be so painful that they are suppressed and eventually bring about physical illness.

The following stories illustrate the way Sarah, Jim and Brian eventually found their own ways to meet the challenge of their illnesses. They show how it is possible to lead fulfilling, productive lives despite recurring problems and setbacks over many years.

Sarah: taking the initiative

Sarah suffers from MS which she has had for 21 years. The onset was sudden and followed a bitter breakdown of her marriage. She was left with a son to bring up on her own. He is now grown up and well established in his own life and career.

Sarah has weakness in both legs which makes walking difficult for her. The weakness started first in her left leg but after about four years it affected both legs.

Once she had been diagnosed, with her deterioration becoming obvious, Sarah's family urged her to take some action as the medical profession seemed to be offering no solutions to her problems. A lot of energy and money was spent seeking a cure, even to the extent of travelling over 200 miles to a clinic which purported to have discovered an 'elixir' to cure the condition. The failure of this 'elixir' to have any impact on her condition left her and the family devastated, angry and severely out of pocket.

In the early stages of any disease people are likely to cast around for a cure, believing that someone, somewhere, must have the answer to their problems. It is so easy, when· you are in shock, to grasp at straws. At that time, fear plays a big part – fear for the future – and the knowledge that you have a progressive illness adds to this fear. This is something I can relate to. There is a feeling that everything is out of control. 'If things are so bad now what will the future bring?' I can remember saying this many times in the past, and it is an expression used over and over again by those coming for help. This feeling is not only confined to the person with the illness but extends to the family, who may panic and allow their imagination to run riot. The person with the problem, with depleted energy and willpower, may be steered towards solutions which are inappropriate, or may give up altogether. To most of us there is the illness and there is the cure – nothing in-between. Fortunately, as time goes by people normally accept their situation and discover realistic ways of coping.

Sarah found her own way. She is a woman of spirit and when interviewed her inner strength was plain to see. She has found out as much as she can about her problem and what is available insofar as medication and support are concerned. She lives alone and runs her own home, has a full-time job and drives her own car. Now at 60 she has just set up a new business partnership, a clear demonstration of her mental drive and determination not to let her MS limit the things she can do.

Sarah has devised her own fitness regime. She began with practising yoga and Pilates but more recently has been attending a gym where the machines are weighted to suit her fitness levels. I asked her who had suggested she got into exercise. Her emphatic reply was 'Not the medics.' She finds the exercise helps and only wishes she had started much earlier.

At one time physical activity was not advised for people with MS in case symptoms became worse. It is now understood that, as with many chronic illnesses, physical activity can be safe. Not only that, but it can have positive therapeutic benefits. However, before starting an exercise programme, whatever your condition, do seek the guidance of a physical therapist. Research supports the part physical activity plays in rehabilitation and demonstrates the resulting improvements in muscle power, mobility, mood, general conditioning and quality of life. It seems that Sarah has acted wisely and sensibly in working on her own rehabilitation programme. Her experience is a clear demonstration that people are quite capable of understanding what is right for them and taking steps to manage things for themselves without professional help. I am not suggesting that everyone should be left alone to get on with things, but where a person demonstrates a capacity for self-management then that should be acknowledged and encouraged.

Current research suggests that patients with MS and other chronic illnesses are best helped by a wide-ranging multi-disciplinary approach, so I asked Sarah if she had been recommended to try other means of help. She said she has never been given any advice on the benefits of relaxation, nor has she ever received any psychotherapy, hypnotherapy or meditation.

We discussed medication and she explained that she gets some benefit from LDN (Low Dose Naltrexone) when she can get it. The drug is licensed only for drug addicts in the UK but studies in America indicate its efficacy in 98 per cent of those taking part in trials of the drug with MS patients. It appears to be effective in reducing spasticity and fatigue and is claimed to be effective in repairing damage to the immune system.

Jim: living with diabetes

Jim was 19 when he was challenged by diabetes. He was an extremely fit young man, playing football and cricket to a very high standard. At the time he was an apprentice engineer working with heavy machinery. He attributed the onset of his illness to the shock of a near miss when an enormous machine broke free of its moorings. As you can imagine, he faced the prospect of his illness having a devastating impact on the most important aspects of his life.

After a period of medical investigations, work on stabilizing his metabolism and training to administer his insulin injections, he was left to pick up the pieces of his life. He had thought he might have to give up his chosen work because of the dangers of being near heavy machinery, but his spirits were lifted when his company offered him a post in the drawing office. Over the years he progressed, becoming a designer, and eventually was promoted to a senior management position. Now, having retired, he is still on a retainer to act as an engineering consultant.

But Jim's path has not been without its pitfalls.

Having been reassured by his employers, Jim set out to pick up the pieces of other areas of his life. He was keen to get back to the sports field. Believing, like most young people, in his own invincibility, he went straight out on to the football field and with very little training took part in a furiously fought cup tie followed by a night out with his team-mates, as was their custom. The result was that before the evening was over he collapsed and was rushed off to hospital.

Jim was fortunate that he was engaged to a very devoted and level-headed young woman. Wendy fully supported his doctor's recommendations that he should make some changes to his lifestyle. She recognized intuitively that Jim was in denial – a reaction common to people who suddenly find themselves faced with extremely challenging, possibly life-threatening situations. These situations immediately threaten people's ability to feel in control and their denial somehow allows them to go on feeling that nothing has changed, even though their behaviour is detrimental to their well-being. If the denial persists and the person is unable to accept the reality of the situation, disastrous results can follow. It shows much for Wendy's intelligence and persuasive persistence that she was able to get Jim to face reality and plan constructively.

Between them Jim and Wendy agreed that football and drinking were not his best friends. As Jim had always been a keen table tennis player, he decided to concentrate on that sport, along with cricket in the summer. Jim had many hairy moments in his attempts to get some balance into his life because he had difficulty resisting Saturday night drinking sessions with his old mates. It was only when he and Wendy eventually married that he settled down and his illness ceased to dominate his life.

However, Jim has always had a stubborn streak and this, combined with his early training that he should never eat between meals, has caused problems from time to time, even though he knows it is necessary to keep his sugar level balanced. He feels it unnecessary to carry some carbohydrate with him, whether he is going to work or for a walk, so he has often been found getting into a hypoglycaemic state (when his sugar levels were too low) and being extremely uncooperative as a result. For a time he had to take a back seat at work because this was happening when he was with important clients. Even on holiday he would insist on completing a long walk in the heat of the day rather than pausing to take essential refreshment. Wendy was always fully alert to this and risked his cross words by gently insisting he ate one of the biscuits she always carried in her handbag. In spite of this – or perhaps thanks to Wendy's understanding – Jim and Wendy have had 38 years of successful marriage, bringing up a family of three children.

Jim's story shows just how easy it is to sabotage essential medical treatment and advice, especially in the early days of adjusting to an illness. It is understandable that Jim, who was 19 when the illness started and full of youthful rebellion, should feel angry that such a serious condition was threatening his career, his future plans and his life.

Wendy played a great part in Jim's healing and his positive adjustment. He was lucky that his healing was helped by his employers, who recognized and used his abilities to the full. Jim has kept active and still plays cricket for his local team 40 years after his diagnosis with Type 1 diabetes. For him it is the perfect game. It doesn't make too many demands physically and the tea-break is a chance to replenish his intake.

Brian: quite a different story

Brian, a veteran of World War II D-Day landings, suffered many privations during his war service and was demobbed in 1945 with a stomach ulcer. He was given pheno-barbitone tablets and advised to go on a completely bland diet and to give up alcohol and cigarettes, and it was also suggested that he should seek light work.

For many reasons he ignored most of the advice and got rid of the tablets. He was determined he would not give up alcohol: he was an expert darts and snooker player, and at that time drinking was very much a part of the pub games scene. Giving up alcohol would mean not just giving up friends but also missing contacts who could offer him casual work, which he did in addition to his job as a heavy goods driver. Much of this work involved pick and spade and hods of bricks. He had a family of four children who adored him and he was determined they should have the best of everything, whatever the cost. He devised his own plan for coping with his ulcer and begged a surgeon to remove the ulcerated part of his stomach, a common operation in the 1950s and 1960s. This drastic treatment seems to have been successful. He continued to live a full life, working most of the time at two jobs and always willing to do favours for others; even after he reached retirement age, he continued to work as a supervisor in a leisure centre for another ten years. He died recently at the age of 93!

Your plan for healing
PART 1

Self-management of chronic illness

As Sarah and Jim's stories illustrate, if you have chronic illness you are in for a marathon rather than a sprint. Marathons need special planning and training, and even super-athletes may 'hit the wall' from time to time before they can claim success. It takes a great deal of psychological and emotional strength and resilience to cope over many years with a long-term and possibly debilitating condition with symptoms that need to be managed on a daily basis. Anyone with a chronic illness will be familiar with the added burdens of pain, exhaustion from sleepless nights, changing and possibly deteriorating physical ability and appearance, poor mobility, tiredness, fear and anxiety.

It is no wonder that self-esteem and confidence take a hammering, especially if the person is no longer the main breadwinner or equal partner in the family economy. Many of the people I have worked with have been particularly sensitive about their diminished role within the family, feeling that their partners or children do not respect them. Added to this loss of self-esteem is a strong feeling of guilt that they are not sharing essential everyday tasks.

It seems to be common practice for employers to find a replacement and dismiss an employee who is not 100 per cent physically fit and able to hold down a full-time job. This can happen within a very few weeks, so money worries are added to the anxiety levels. Ideally it should be possible for employer and employee to sit down together and work out ways in which the job and hours could be adjusted so that each gains mutual benefit from the arrangement. When an employee is lost to a company, valuable knowledge skills and experience are also lost. However, it can take months to get a specialist appointment and even longer to complete tests before a full diagnosis of the condition is made, and by that time the wheels of industry and commerce have rolled on.

In my own case, although the university was extremely

understanding about my situation and kept my job open for 12 months, it was fully two years before I had a diagnosis, and at that stage, without having had any treatment, I was in no fit state physically or psychologically to go back to teaching. I was unable to drive (or even sit in the car), I could not concentrate to read or write and my days were dominated by pain. None of my medical advisers would venture an opinion on a date when I could return to work. Like many others with chronic conditions, I was suffering from the consequences of my illness and the isolation it brought with it. Some action was called for – but what? All I knew at that time was that it would be fatal to drift into a state of helplessness because that is a prelude to depression. In my mind was the image of myself at the age of four or five visiting my elderly paternal grandfather, who spent his days lounging on a chaise longue, a common piece of living-room furniture in those days over 70 years ago. I was told he had been an invalid for years. I did not want that to be my fate.

This is when the seed of the plan was sown in my mind. It is only since I began to write this book that I realize that my quest for healing started much earlier than my experience with Helen on the pain management course. You may recall instances in your own life that might be defined as healing experiences. They may not bring any permanent or significant change for the better but they may be just enough to lift you out of some dark place. Some people draw their strength from their religious beliefs and the power of prayer, others may be inspired by the experience of others who have overcome their difficulties. Healing experiences do not have to be dramatic. They can stem from a chance remark, a chance meeting, a conversation with a stranger, a well-loved piece of music, a favourite poem or a good book, something on the TV or radio. It is so easy to overlook, as I did, events that are significant healing points or staging posts in your personal transformation. The following account illustrates this point.

My first task was to get back control of my life even though the medics had formed no treatment plan by that time. I had by now taken early retirement on sickness grounds and received a lump sum which relieved some of my financial worries. Around this time I was approached by a political party to see if I would be interested in standing as a candidate in the forthcoming local election. Party politics had no appeal for me, but in any case I was in no condition to think of any work outside the house. Acknowledging that I was now almost completely housebound and heading for a permanent position on the sofa made me realize how isolated I had become.

This realization was enough to rekindle, maybe only faintly at that time, my fighting spirit. It was a critical point that stimulated me to plan for the future.

Planning for the future is one of the most healthy and uplifting activities you can do. I was interested in what was going on in our village, which had been my family home for many generations and which, although much enlarged, had lost its heart. Like many others over the years, it had lost its shops apart from a post office and convenience store. It was no longer self-sufficient. A common complaint was that it was no longer possible to buy a ball of wool in the village, and it was necessary to travel into town, eight miles away, to buy anything other than groceries.

By chance, a near-derelict property came up for sale next to the post office, just a few hundred yards from my home. As it was affordable, with the encouragement of my family I decided to buy the property, get builders in to renovate it and convert it into a wool, craft and hobbies shop. The type of shop was influenced by the female members of my immediate and extended family, who were in touch with the Women's Institute, Young Wives, mothers with children in local schools and pensioners' groups. I had nothing but encouragement from the village population when they heard that a new shop was opening. The shop would become a focal point, a meeting place, not only for a gossip but a place where people could exchange ideas on their hobbies and learn new skills.

I was a knight in three-ply armour! At once I felt back in control of my own destiny. I had taken some action that restored my self-respect and I had something to aim for. I had the added benefit of knowing I had contributed to the well-being of other people.

My role in the enterprise was to oversee the finances, meet salesmen and order stock. I had to rely on others to do the physical work of dealing with customers, keeping the place clean and stocking shelves. I felt so much better!

My triumph was short-lived, however, as a collapse soon after the shop opened meant my admission to hospital and a decision to operate for the removal of a spinal tumour. The results of the operation brought about problems that meant that my struggle for healing became even more difficult. I felt that I had lost all the benefit I had gained so far, and physically I was even worse than I had been at the start of my illness. My emotional and psychological well-being suffered as my pain increased and my mobility became more limited.

My plan for healing evolved slowly following my experience on the pain management course. It developed as I worked as a therapist on the course and I had the opportunity to undertake further training in psychotherapy and hypnotherapy. I was able to learn more about pain and its treatment as a result of being involved with the pain management team at the University of Washington Hospital in Seattle. The more I learned, the more convinced did I become that I could not make myself solely dependent on other people for healing. This had to come from within because all the medical profession could offer me were painkillers and other drugs to which I was allergic and which might result in life-threatening consequences. As far as I could see, it was self-help or nothing.

It took a long time to work out a coherent plan that would eventually lead me towards a point where I could honestly say, 'I am back in control of my life, I am no longer a slave to my illness, I am feeling better and what's more I am progressing towards improved health every day.' I know that a major contribution to my ability to cope came from helping others with painful illnesses, either through face-to-face therapy or through my writing. There is no time to feel ill when you are fully involved with people or have deadlines to meet!

Self-management of chronic illness

In recent years, self-management of chronic illness has been actively encouraged and reinforced by educational programmes designed to help people take more control of their illnesses. The research evidence, and my own experience in designing and running such programmes, suggests that when people take responsibility for their own care there are more positive results than when they are merely passive recipients of treatment.

Although healing may be enhanced with greater 'patient control', circumstances may limit your ability to take control. Housing conditions, income, family circumstances and work demands, psychological and emotional factors and, of course, the severity of disablement produced by the illness may make things difficult, but do not be tempted to give up trying. You cannot neglect your illness because of what else is going on in your life any more than you can allow your illness to dominate your life to the exclusion of all else.

Molly, aged 48, an unmarried woman who was severely asthmatic, struggled with both her own illness and that of her disabled father, who needed 24-hour care. The situation was not resolved until she experienced a crisis in her own health which led to an emergency hospital admission. Fortunately the crisis resulted in help and support from medical and social services which relieved her of providing full-time care for her father. At that point she was able to start taking care of her own health and pick up the threads of a long-neglected social life. She used her newfound freedom to return to study, following part-time courses at her local college, and to undertake a fitness programme. She is now thinking of a return to work. She has a much more relaxed relationship with her father now that she is relieved of the anxiety of his full-time care.

Self-management must include self-monitoring

In order to take charge of your illness you must be in touch at all times with your body, mind and feelings and the way you are getting on with others. You need to question yourself constantly about the way you treat yourself. Are you overeating, drinking to excess, getting too tired, lounging about too much, shunning company, being inflexible and failing to accept and adapt to your new situation? Are you sticking to your medical regime, which is essential for your well-being? Are you following your exercise and relaxation programmes? This process of self-monitoring is important if you are to understand and cope with setbacks, which are inevitable for anyone with chronic illness. It is particularly important if you find that all the progress you have made in combating your condition seems suddenly to have disappeared for no apparent reason, something that happens to many of us who have chronic pain, fibromyalgia or ME. Self-management must include learning what causes your setbacks and how to avoid them.

As the book progresses I aim to help you understand this process and to show you ways to follow it through from day to day.

The following plan is designed to help you cope to the best of your ability.

1

Accept you have an illness

Accepting that you have an illness is a vital stage in getting back in control of your symptoms and your life. You have to strike a balance between being completely at the mercy of your illness and giving up on everything life has to offer, and the rather extreme form of denial that I seem to have indulged in. I was probably a workaholic, taking on more work than was good for me, thinking the world would fall apart if I took time out. I carried work on into my leisure time, which was already packed with activity, having three children who needed to be ferried around to sports and musical activities. My evenings were filled with amateur theatricals, rehearsals and teaching life-saving. Even when my illness became apparent I tended to push it aside and carry on to the point of exhaustion, resulting in excessive stress and even more devastating symptoms. Seeking help with anything I did was a low priority for me. To ask for help in my case was to acknowledge a weakness and accept that I was really sick and no longer in control. To admit to illness was to admit defeat.

I do not think I am alone in responding to illness in this way. Indeed, denial seems to be a common response to chronic illness. I have worked with many pain patients who make no concessions to the fact that they have a severely disabling condition and continue to throw themselves into activities that they did when they were fit.

Fred, for example, who was on a pain management course, spent his weekend changing the engine in his car (is this a one-man job for anybody?). The result was he was laid up for a week. He was a great exponent of the 'crash and burn' approach to therapy.

Denial can result in making a bad situation much worse. Acceptance is the first stage in your progress towards a good quality of life, but accepting your condition does not mean being fatalistic, curling up and allowing things to happen to you. It means accepting the reality of your situation and working around it. Anyone with an addiction or mental health problem will know that they will make no progress until they have come to terms fully with their condition. Anyone with chronic heart disease will never cope with the rigours of a healthy diet unless they fully accept the nature of their illness.

In the case of diabetes, anything but wholehearted acceptance on the part of the person means that self-management alone is a vain hope, as there is a need for lifelong discipline and coopera- tion with health professionals. With good management there is no reason why any person with diabetes should not have a good, fulfilling life. Good management requires accepting guidance on what to eat, when and how much, and taking exercise and how much. It requires keeping checks on blood sugar, blood pressure and cholesterol levels, and having regular attention to feet, heart, kidneys, eyes, teeth and gums. A recent government report indi- cates that many people are missing out on these checks, suggesting there is a lack of communication between the medical services and those at risk.

This breakdown is costly for the National Health Service (NHS) but even more so for the individual. Poor self-management can lead, over time, to deterioration because of an accumulation of blood sugar, resulting in heart disease, heart attacks, strokes, kidney disease, nerve damage, digestive problems, eye disease or tooth and gum problems. If these problems arise, there will be a need for emergency treatment, hospitalization, life-saving inter- vention, amputations and further medication. If these fail then of course there is a risk of death. No matter how good the medical services, the person with diabetes has to accept the condition and with it the responsibility for self-management using the support of the professionals.

Acceptance can take time and may not take place until the person with chronic illness has been able to recognize and face up to everything that has been lost as a result of the illness. These losses can include loss of physical prowess, control over bodily functions, loss of a positive body image, loss of work, loss of status, income and independence . . . you can probably think of so many more to add to the list. Such losses are hard to deal with. Some ill- nesses bring with them a succession of losses that occur from time to time, and the process of acceptance has to start all over again.

Growing older brings loss of a number of abilities but at least an older person has had time to prepare mentally and has probably had the satisfaction of living a reasonably active life beforehand. When chronic illness strikes before a person has had time to flourish or when that person is at his or her peak, the emotional impact is very powerful. Losing your health can be as devastating in its impact as losing someone very close to you and, just as when you lose someone very close to you, it is important that you have time to grieve and feel sorry for yourself. The duration of this process is not fixed but varies with each person. Nevertheless, it must be experienced before you can accept everything that is involved in your illness and move on to taking positive action on your own behalf. Grieving and acceptance may be particularly difficult for some people and may never be achieved satisfactorily without professional help. Unless these stages are accomplished, treatment for the illness is unlikely to have much impact and it can take a long time for the healing process to begin.

Begin the process by learning to recognize when you are in denial and failing to face up to a problem. Learn to recognize when you are overdoing things, becoming over-anxious, feeling low, indulging in self-defeating negative thoughts. Above all, listen to your body. Your body signals it is in trouble by an increase in pain and fatigue, digestive and bowel problems, headaches, palpitations, muscle weakness or a worsening of the symptoms of your illness. All these are the means your mind and body have of communicating that there are rough times not far away and that it is time to take swift action.

2

Take action

A lot of time, energy and money can be wasted seeking a cure for your illness. This leads only to disappointment, and each disappointment is harder to cope with than the one before. During the time I have spent researching this book I have encountered a number of websites eager to point out the benefits of following a specific course of action to bring about a cure for any number of chronic illnesses. They are very slick in their presentation, drawing you in, listing endorsement after endorsement from people saying how much their condition has improved – and all the time you are being invited to make that final click of your mouse that commits you to spending several hundred pounds on a 'cure' that may be worthless. The internet has become the modern equivalent of the fairground, with numerous quack doctors whose sole purpose is to relieve you of your money. It is a problem to pick out the genuine and authentic remedies, so beware! The longer your search goes on with no positive outcome, the worse your pain, feelings of depression and the illness itself will seem. The longer the process lasts, the greater the fear. It is easy to forget how it feels to be healthy.

Human beings have an innate capacity to change. It is this capacity that helps us to 'dig ourselves out of a hole'. You no doubt remember occasions in your own life when you have used your grit and determination to overcome difficulties. Illness can have the effect of dampening down your inner strengths, but they are still there. You have to ask yourself how much you want to change. For some, the changes required may seem overwhelming, but this book is intended to show you how it is possible to move forward, to help you decide what things you can do to get better and to help you commit time and energy to the process. Getting better means thought, commitment and appropriate action.

When we take one step towards recovery it is easier to take the next, and the next. Each step takes you to a different place from which you will gain a new perspective and see more opportunities for getting better. However, as you take more responsibility for your own healing you need to be prepared for perhaps fundamental changes in the way you think, how you see yourself and the goals you set. You may even change the way you conduct your relationships. This happens to everyone as circumstances change throughout life.

Such changes are part of a natural progression, but in times of crisis such as the death of a loved one, divorce, illness or the loss of a job change is forced upon us and that is not so easy to cope with. These events suddenly take away much of our ability to make choices and we may be pushed along by events. Crises of this kind lead us to strive to regain what we have lost. In the case of long-term illness, it seems that the more you strive, the more difficult is the task of achieving real healing. For months, perhaps years, I was obsessed with getting back to my job as a teacher and doing all the things with the family that I had done before – Sunday morning football, swimming, life-saving club, brass band practice and concerts, acting and singing. As my ability to do these things became just a memory, so my sense of loss, my anger, my feelings of hopelessness and helplessness became greater. With healing, my life took quite a new direction.

Action involves making choices

Passivity is your worst enemy. Make the decision to take some action to help yourself. Making that decision and acting on it will give you a great sense of power that may have been missing from your life for a very long time.

Virtually everything we do in life involves making a choice. We do not always have complete freedom of choice. Most of us find choice is limited by factors such as available cash, competition with others for jobs, responsibility for others and, of course, ability.

You may not be responsible for your illness but you are responsible for the way you manage it. If you have chronic illness your ability will be limited but you owe it to yourself to do the best you can. Sometimes it appears easier to settle for your present position, to drift and allow things to happen to you. I have had to face up to these thoughts on more than one occasion when nothing I do seems to makes a difference to my illness or the way I am coping. If you find yourself feeling like this, remind yourself that any choice, any change you make is entirely up to you. If you decide not to take action, so be it: but there are always new avenues to explore, many new choices you can make. Decide *now* to take control over as many aspects of your life as possible. Make a start by keeping a daily diary, recording:

- the time you get up in the morning;
- the time you go to bed;
- how long you spend lounging in an armchair, sofa or bed during the day;
- how long you spend watching TV or on your computer or games console;
- how long you spend on exercise, including your normal household tasks;
- how long you spend on hobbies or handicrafts or socializing outside your home;
- how long you spend commuting to work;
- how long you spend at work;
- how long you spend on work you bring home.

Decide whether you need to take some action to reallocate your time differently.

Take account of whether your review of your lifestyle indicates you are active enough, isolated or inclined to shun social contact, or whether your travelling and work activity is out of balance with your leisure time and is putting too much stress in your life.

If you work or look after the family you can choose to organize things differently, especially if you think you are indispensable or making a martyr of yourself. Remember, the quickest way to make a chronic illness worse is to allow yourself to become exhausted.

Write a list of the different areas of your life, noting where you have some choice in determining how you manage from day to day. You might conclude that the only way to cope is to make a series of major changes, and people often do this. They change jobs, house, countries, even husbands or wives in an effort to alter life for the better. Such changes can be made from sheer desperation, and if not thought through they can have serious consequences. The prospect of making any change may seem overwhelming to you at this time, but let's make it simple.

- You can choose what time you get up in the morning and what time you go to bed. (If you have got into the habit of lying in bed till midday or later because you have nothing better to do, or because you stay up late watching TV or DVDs or having a few too many 'nightcaps', then it is time to think about change.)
- You can choose what to wear.
- You can choose what and when to eat.

- You can choose when you go out.
- You can choose where you go and who you meet.

The idea of making choices is a very simple one. Virtually everything we do calls for a choice to be made. People who are unable to make a choice or have their choices taken away from them because of poverty, disabling illness or being confined at Her Majesty's pleasure have little chance to grow and develop or make anything of their lives. So start by thinking of the choices you *can* make. Above all, you can choose to take the first steps towards making a change that involves you becoming an expert in your own illness, a choice that involves you taking the lead in your progress towards self-management and healing.

Once you have decided to take action to enhance your well-being and to follow the path of self-healing, you need to be determined, plan, persist and above all enjoy the work involved. You are the only one who can put a brake on achieving the rewards. Once you have made the choice you may be surprised at just how many people will be there to help you reach your goals.

Seek information

To make the best choices you can, you need to find out as much as possible about your illness. It will help you to know how it will progress, what treatments are available, both conventional and complementary, and what steps you can take to reduce its impact on your life. Do not be afraid to ask your doctor for information and help. So, make sure you book a double appointment when you want to talk about your condition. If you have questions or concerns about your health or your treatment, be sure to write them down before you see the doctor. Many people get confused or overawed when entering the surgery and forget what they came for or phrase things clumsily.

If you are not happy with the way your doctor responds to questions, or if he or she deals with you impatiently, then you must consider whether this doctor is the right one for you. Your relationship could potentially last many years. If there are a number of GPs in the practice, find out whether one of them is particularly knowledgeable about your condition.

When you have a chronic illness it is important to have a meeting with your doctor at least once a year to review the progress of your illness and the medication prescribed. I have found it helpful – and I am sure my GP has too – to write down the history of my illness and its treatment over the years, as I see it, then hand it to the doctor for comment as a start to the discussion. Writing things down will provide you and your GP with a focus for the consultation and will ensure you do not forget to mention anything that concerns you. You cannot expect a busy GP to remember every detail about you and your treatment, especially in a large medical centre. Your doctor will be able to correct any facts or misconceptions that you may have and offer reassurance if you are getting things out of proportion. Take the opportunity during the discussion to explore any possible new avenues of treatment or to present your own ideas for action that you might take on your own behalf to aid your well-being.

Some surgeries now employ a pharmacist to advise on medication and to carry out the all-important reviews. Take the opportunity to discuss whether your medication is having a real impact on your condition or is adding to your burden by producing side effects out of proportion to the benefits you are receiving.

Be wary of being given additional medication to counteract any side effects you are experiencing. Remember, long-term use of medication, even though it may not seem to be producing bad side effects in the short term, may with long-term use have very serious implications for you. This is particularly important when you are prescribed a cocktail of drugs. Use the internet, if you have access to it, for information about the drugs you are on, paying attention to their efficacy and possible side effects.

The internet is a good source of reference; if you or a member of your family have a computer this will help you to access much more information. Some of the information is highly technical, but you will find with experience that there are many websites prepared especially for people with chronic illness. These can lead you into many sources of help and advice. You will find the personal accounts inspiring and you will discover quickly what has helped other people in their quest for healing. You may find that using the internet provides a connection to other people and groups who can offer support.

3

Make use of support

Get connected

Like me, you may have had an upbringing that stressed independence as a desirable quality and asking for help as a sign of weakness. It is a virtue to find the answers to your own problems and to carry out tasks unaided. However, we live in a society where everybody is mutually dependent, where no one can survive in isolation. We are nurtured in family groups, educated together with others, eat food produced by the collective efforts of others and have to rely on the cooperation of many to provide places of work, play and worship.

A healthy, happy person is one who is able to love and to work. Self-worth and happiness come from the way we relate to others, the way they relate to us, and our ability to perform some task that brings us rewards – financial, social and emotional. Illness strikes at our ability to achieve these ends and we can easily become isolated. When you are ill, your view of yourself can easily become distorted: you can easily view yourself as a victim, with little power, believing that your place in the world of work, family and the community has become diminished. At this point you become separated emotionally, and sometimes physically, from the world of work, the family and social relationships. You need to cling on to an idea of your own self-worth, as a person with an illness that limits but does not nullify your abilities, your relationships or your inherent strengths and weaknesses. In this case, the goal of healing must centre on you as a person and your need to develop an appreciation of yourself as still remaining a valuable part of your network of social relationships. Your work connections may have gone permanently, and with them your own sense of having some status. You may have to adjust to remaining isolated from the world of work, and it may take time to find something to take its place.

Stay connected

Healthy relationships are the foundation for good health, well-being and healing. If problems arise and the going gets tough, relationships and mutual support can be instrumental in helping you return to normal, regain equilibrium and strengthen your ability to bounce back from crises. People who isolate themselves from others and 'pull up the drawbridge' or build walls around themselves have an impoverished emotional life. Sometimes people living closely with others in the family can cut themselves off emotionally from their loved ones, often causing problems for themselves and those around them. This is often a sign that depression has set in and other family members may also begin to show signs of depression, or there may be evidence that the family is becoming dysfunctional. Relationships may break down altogether. Many surveys indicate that people enjoying good supportive family relationships cope better with long-term illness than those who do not have close family support. Health practitioners need to be alert to this with a view to suggesting appropriate sources of alternative help.

How do you relate to others?

Your illness may lead to you feeling remote from friends and family so you may have unconsciously changed the way you react to them.

Take a step back and observe yourself in action.

Do you respond to them with a grunt? Or with words such as 'What do you think?' or 'What do you expect?' so commonly used in our favourite soaps. These are abrupt and aggressive put-downs designed to cut off normal conversation and do nothing to oil the wheels of social intercourse. Do you have any real conversation at all? Do you find yourself habitually criticizing the behaviour or achievements of your spouse or children? Do you ever give whole-hearted unambiguous praise or is it always tempered by a sting in the tail? Of course, we have all met someone who is perfectly healthy who behaves in such boorish ways but if you value your relationships you will need to avoid this form of behaviour.

If you do find yourself slipping into this off-hand means of communication then for a week undertake this exercise.

Positive communication

Initiate conversation, especially to ask about the welfare of others. Listen to whatever the other person wishes to say. If you have not seen someone for some time, start by asking for news of the family – his or her partner's welfare, children's achievements, plans for holidays. Whenever you are in conversation find something complimentary to say about the other person – how well he or she is looking or, if you notice something different such as a new hairstyle, say how attractive it looks. Show equal concern to your partner. Take particular care with your children, especially if you have got into the habit of snapping at them, criticizing them, finding fault. Try to eliminate that behaviour for the whole week and try to praise as many things as you can. They might think you have lost it, but you will find there is a different atmosphere about the house and they will take it as a sign that you are feeling better. Changing your behaviour in this way is one of the most effective means of promoting your own healing because you will find that other people become much more positive in the way they relate to you. Just think about it . . .

Mark

Mark suffered from spondylitis for many years. He had a job which involved driving for long hours; when he got home at night he was in pain and exhausted and all he wanted to do was withdraw from the family situation. This was difficult in a small house with two children, a talkative wife and a TV permanently switched on! In order to cope, he consumed painkillers and anti-inflammatory tablets – and a number of cans of beer. His long-suffering wife tolerated this for a number of years before her patience wore thin and the couple became estranged in the same house. The atmosphere was always tense and when the children became of age they left home. As soon as the second child had left home for university the couple realized there was nothing keeping them together. Mark's wife sought company outside the home and this became a real bone of contention. It was not long before Mark accused her of having an affair, which resulted in his wife walking out.

Mark immediately put the house up for sale and moved into rented accommodation. Living alone, his depression was a matter for concern to his employers. He was having many days off complaining of back pain and the adverse effects of driving. He was given notice that he was unreliable and it was costing too much to cover for his absences. To his painkillers were added antidepressants, on which he became dependent.

By now his only income was incapacity benefit and debts built up. To his pain and depression were added obesity and high blood pressure. He was in a downward spiral, making excuses for failing to keep in touch with his family. He would not invite them into his home. To their credit, his children persisted in continuing the relationship even though they felt very upset at what they saw as rejection. They went on caring and refused to be put off, continuing to phone and making a point of inviting him to family functions and celebrations.

It took about five years and the birth of a couple of grandchildren to bring them closer. As the relationships developed, he became more involved with his children and their families and began to show signs of change. He started to look at his weight problem and made changes to his diet. He badgered his doctor to review his long-term use of painkillers and anti-depressants. Eventually he took up model-making, something he had enjoyed at school. He became engrossed in the hobby and joined a local group who shared his interest. Through this he became much more confident at mixing with other people, joining in their conversation and sharing his expertise.

Today, Mark appreciates that being with other people is the key to his well-being, and he knows that leading a life of isolation has been very destructive. He is adamant that he will never again build a wall around himself. He is eager to find ways of returning to part-time work.

Accepting help is not always easy

Seeking help in any situation does not always come easily, and many of us hesitate to accept help even when the simplest of problems arise. Yet we know that when we do seek or accept help, any feelings of reluctance soon disappear as the problem is resolved. We have no trouble or inhibitions about making offers of help, but when we become ill we are often reluctant to seek help other than initial medical intervention. We have already discussed the issue of accepting that we have an illness and the problems this can bring. It is often very difficult to take the next step, from acceptance to admitting we need help and setting out to get it.

Chronic illness reduces our capacity to help ourselves in all sorts of ways, and we often prefer to put up with the problem and carry on regardless, trusting that things will sort themselves out eventually. Fortunately, many of us have families and colleagues who show concern, who can see the devastation the illness brings and who offer good advice and share the load. Failure to ask for help or refusal to accept it when offered can increase the sense of isolation and bad relationships.

Sometimes we are reluctant to accept that things we once did very easily are now beyond our capacity – for example, mowing the lawn, making beds, hoovering, small DIY jobs, shopping, all of which can bring on fatigue and pain. Yet we push on to the point of exhaustion, never dreaming to ask for help even though we know the consequences. Pushing on without support means that there is no fuel left in the tank to do anything for the rest of the day, let alone acknowledge and meet the needs of other people who depend on us for emotional or physical support.

Working on without help in this way destroys any chance we have of managing our illness successfully and getting to a point when we feel there is some balance in our lives. It is the complete antithesis of healing. Accepting help, and feeling and showing gratitude for that help, can do much to bring about healing. You get a lot of emotional support from knowing that someone cares enough about you and understands your needs.

Anyone who has diabetes will find it difficult to survive without support from many people as the illness needs a high degree of technical knowledge and skill for its management. Support is essential from a large team of health professionals, including GPs, practice nurses, dietitians, psychologists, pharmacists, exercise specialists, dentists, eye, foot, kidney and heart specialists and maybe social workers.

Healing can come from helping others

In the early stages of an illness being altruistic is probably low down on the list of anyone's priorities, but as symptoms and feelings become more controlled, doing something to help others can help the healing process. The experience of healing can have a strong emotional impact. Restored physical abilities, emotional energy and a re-ignited spirit, combined with a sense of gratitude, can lead to a very strong desire to give something back to others. Many of the patients who benefited from being on the pain management programme at Walton Hospital in Liverpool, myself included, wanted to know how they could get involved in helping others in pain. Research shows that giving to others can be rewarding and can be seen as a healing activity.

Doing something for others need not demand great skills or be very glamorous. I once belonged to an operatic society where an elderly lady turned up at rehearsals week after week to make tea for the performers. She had severe arthritis and claimed that being alongside the singers, making the tea and doing little jobs for them made her feel so much better, eased her pain and was the highlight of her week. Martin Seligman, who researches in the field of positive psychology and writes about optimism and achieving happiness, maintains that doing things for others as a matter of routine has the effect of producing a feeling of happiness. Why not try giving way to people in traffic and enjoy the smile they give you!

Many simple everyday gestures of goodwill such as this count for a lot.

Make use of support groups

There can be very few people who have grown up without coming under the influence of groups – families or family substitutes, school, college, church, youth clubs, work teams, sports teams, the list is endless. They are responsible for our nurture: learning about relationships, about giving and receiving, ideas of right and wrong, stimulating thought, creativity and discussion, and, of course, having fun! Throughout my professional life I have had experience of working with therapeutic groups. I have been involved with leadership or therapeutic roles with young offenders, isolated and depressed housewives, dysfunctional families, families in crisis, disturbed children and adolescents and their carers, and people with chronic pain and various other chronic illnesses. As a result I can honestly say that the group is a powerful source, not only of nurture, education, information and friendship, but of healing.

Some years ago I was asked to work with a group of teachers and carers in a school for disturbed adolescents. My brief was to help the staff learn skills that they could use in their day-to-day work with the children. It soon became apparent that the group members were incapable of focusing on the topic and that the group was full of tension. There was a feeling that no one could understand what it felt like to be a teacher entering a room where the children were so disturbed they could not focus on learning or any other activity.

Gradually, each member of the group was able to talk about his or her intense feelings of fear, anxiety and complete inadequacy when facing the children. As people disclosed their feelings it became obvious that their colleagues were hearing things from each other that they had never heard before. Everyone assumed that their colleagues were coping very well and that they were the only ones who were not. It took a great deal of courage for individuals to confess their lack of confidence and their fears about the consequences of being unable to control young adults whose behaviour was, to say the least, unpredictable. Once the fears had been expressed, the teachers began to focus positively on ways in which they could provide emotional and professional support for each other.

Over the ensuing weeks they devised a plan for sharing information about approaches that worked and did not work with the youngsters. In the course of the sessions I had introduced some relaxation techniques that I was in the habit of using with people with pain. The teachers found these extremely helpful personally and the techniques did much to restore confidence in their work. Several teachers decided to introduce relaxation into their classroom work before getting down to academic studies. The results they reported back were truly remarkable as the behaviour of the children was completely transformed.

So, make a point of finding out about support groups in your area for people with your condition. You can discover helpful information about the illness and how to manage it from others who share your difficulties. Fellow members can inspire you to try new ways of coping as you seek new solutions to your problems. Quite apart from this, you can gain much needed emotional support and maybe even become a tower of strength to others in the group. You have to remember that those people with your illness are the 'experts' and together you share a vast amount of information and experience. Your support group can be a source of healing, perhaps even the most important one you will have.

If you belong to a therapeutic or support group you have the potential to have several 'therapists' rather than just one. Because a group has a membership of people who are at different stages in their illness you can observe and be inspired by the stories they have about their own journey towards improved health. You will also have experience of other people making changes – sometimes dramatic changes – in their lives, and this can be extremely encouraging for you to continue your own healing plan. A group that works well together is able to work on the range of physical, mental, emotional and spiritual issues involved in healing.

As a therapist, I always prefer to work with people in a group because the power of the group greatly enhances my work with the patients. There is always someone willing and able to reinforce the message I am giving so that it has a greater impact. Whenever people are finding it difficult to come to terms with their situation or to make essential lifestyle changes, group members help them to overcome their resistance. Therapy often involves facing up to deep-seated emotional issues which can be upsetting and embarrassing. These issues can inhibit a person undergoing one-to-one therapy, but in a group it helps to see other people having the courage to share information and feelings with other members. The individual gains strength from the support of the group members as they face their problems. It must be stressed that the group provides a safe environment for a member to raise issues that cannot be easily discussed within the family.

The group is also vital in giving mutual support to face the future realistically, and of course it plays a major role in boosting self-esteem and confidence and reducing any feelings of isolation.

Information about groups specifically serving the needs of people with your illness can usually be found among the myriad of notices within your local health centre. If you cannot find anything then ask the receptionist. Alternatively, try your local library or your phone book, or if you have a computer you may find it helpful to look at the websites of the various associations and charities relating to your condition. From them you will glean helpful information about the illness and resources available to help you. The websites also show information about support groups throughout the UK. Make use of the information about these resources that I have listed at the end of this book.

Using community resources

This country is rich in its wide provision of opportunities for people to follow social, cultural and artistic interests. These provisions are vital for all sections of the population in maintaining enjoyment and mental and spiritual health. People with chronic illness also need to participate fully in activities that are spiritually enriching. Unfortunately, they are often limited by such things as fatigue, limited concentration and their inability to sit or stand for long periods.

I can speak from experience in an art class, where I was in a group of able-bodied people. My sitting time on upright dining chairs was about five minutes before pain set in, and I needed to move about frequently. I was not able to keep up with the others and my enjoyment of the class was spoiled. I do not think I gained anything from the experience other than deciding not to try again.

Another venture was learning to play guitar. The class was held in a junior school and the only seating was the tiny child-size chairs. You can guess the rest! There is a vital need for social and cultural groups within the community that take into account people's individual needs.

4

Healing needs energy

We have already seen that failure to accept the limitations placed on you by your illness is not helpful. The 'crash and burn' policy means stumbling from one crisis to another, and no progress is made towards getting on top of the illness or working towards a lifestyle that satisfies.

There are two important tasks you can perform to aid your own healing:

- conserving energy
- creating energy (this will be dealt with in 'Your plan for healing – Part 2').

Conserving energy

Conserving energy takes a lot of work – 'thinking work', that is. It was probably the hardest task I had to perform in carrying out my healing plan. Every day, no matter what I did, I seemed to reach a point of exhaustion, often after being up and about for only an hour or two. From talking to people with pain or ME or other chronic illness, this seems to be a common complaint. The obvious thing to do would appear to be to seek rest, to resort to the couch or bed.

Sleep is undoubtedly a very powerful healer. Sleep deprivation, whatever its cause diminishes your capacity not only to heal but to function. In periods of acute illness bed-rest is vital to allow the body to heal itself, but this is not helpful in the long term. Staying in bed for a long time or lounging on a couch without exercise or movement causes loss of stamina and muscle tone. Bones lose their mass and become brittle, the heart and lungs cease to function efficiently and blood flow is reduced. As a result, waste is not completely eliminated. The sorry tale continues: balance is adversely affected and we begin to stumble and fall. This is particularly bad for older people or anyone with arthritis or other spinal condition.

If you have chronic pain, bed-rest is certainly not the answer. Even three days' bed-rest can decrease stamina by 25 per cent, and the longer you remain inactive the harder it is to regain strength. You can easily put on weight and exhaustion sets in more quickly when you try to do things. In this situation depression can soon follow and you enter a downward spiral. Your illness is then likely to deteriorate out of control.

Inactivity leads to brooding and anticipating trouble so you do not feel good. You may feel depressed, dwelling on all the bad things that have happened in the past, obsessed by a constant stream of negative thoughts that drain every last drop of energy; in that condition, healing becomes an impossible dream. Later I shall give you some tips on getting rid of these negative thoughts (see Chapter 9).

In contradiction, Louise Hay, in her book *You Can Heal Your Life* (Hay House Books, latest edition 2004), advocates bed-rest and fasting for days and even weeks to enable the body to use its energy to clear itself of virtually all illness. In the interests of research for this book I spent a weekend, not fasting completely, but living on soups and sugar-free juices. I did not take to my bed but spent my time quietly reading and listening to music. I used my exercise bike for five minutes each day and pottered about the garden. After 72 hours I felt full of energy and pain-free. It is an experience I shall repeat one day but I doubt I shall follow Louise Hay's complete prescription.

Nevertheless, conserving energy is the cornerstone of your progress towards a life that is not dominated by illness, stress and pain. So, how is it done?

Get to know your limitations

Listen to your body

You may find that carrying out certain activities produces discomfort and fatigue, or even makes you short-tempered. You may not be able to sit in a car for very long or undertake long journeys. You may find it difficult to sit upright at your computer or dining table. Shopping in a supermarket may lead to exhaustion and place real limits on your ability to run a home. Even standing in the kitchen preparing a meal or washing up can be an ordeal. These common, everyday activities are the basis of normal, minimal everyday functioning; the inability to cope with them is a real downer and, of course, saps your energy even more.

Energy is the fuel of your healing

Take the time to discover the point where anything you are doing brings you discomfort. That is the time to finish. It is also the benchmark by which you judge your progress towards improved well-being. It may be inconvenient to end an activity so soon, but look upon yourself as being in training. If possible, during this period of training call upon the help of a friend or partner to monitor your efforts. If you carry on too long you may find that exhaustion or pain sets in or – which is worse – your judgement can be affected. A health practitioner who took part in one of my groups confided that when he pushed on beyond his limits he became short-tempered with both patients and staff, and on more than one occasion his concentration failed and mistakes were only averted by the intervention of his practice nurse.

In my own case, I found at one stage I could only drive comfortably for half an hour before pain set in. That was the signal to hand over the driving to my wife. I also found I could peel only four potatoes comfortably, so the easiest thing for me was take potatoes off the menu or have them baked. These limits became the important baselines for me in my quest for conserving energy and subsequently for measuring my progress and finding new solutions to problems.

I have already mentioned the supermarket: if this is a problem for you and you really feel you must shop there then see how long you can manage comfortably. At the point you feel any discomfort, *stop!* Go home and use your energy to enjoy the rest of the day. Most supermarkets have a delivery service available so why not make use of it?

Planning, preparation and pacing

Anyone who has read my book *The Pain Management Handbook* (Sheldon Press, 2011) will be familiar with these three concepts and will be aware that I liken people to a rechargeable battery having a finite store of energy. Carrying out certain tasks or doing them for too long will leave us drained. The more often we drain the battery, the more difficult it will be to achieve any kind of healing. You constantly have to make decisions about the length of time or the physical effort involved in carrying out any task before you need to recharge your battery. So, think ahead and plan, prepare and pace yourself.

Planning involves working out in advance as far as possible what activities you are going to put into your day, thinking what you need to do to carry them out and deciding how you can make things easy for yourself. Abandon all ideas of multi-tasking.

In my early days of recovery I developed a way of getting through my days that allowed me sufficient energy to enjoy an evening with my family. It was no use packing things in during the day and then spending the evening depleted and in pain, having no interest in how the rest of the family had spent their day or having to go to bed at a very early hour.

Showering and getting dressed in the morning took almost two hours and left me very exhausted. After a period of deep relaxation and a cup of tea I went for a short walk with the dog. For the dog's benefit I aimed to reach a certain tree in the field behind my home before returning to do some exercises, after which I started to prepare a light lunch. After lunch I would spend half an hour or so with a good book, by which time the dog was ready for another walk. (It did feel as though I had become the servant and the dog the master – but that can happen when you have a dog. Still, he was good company and it saved me becoming a victim of daytime television!) Then home and a cup of tea before preparing the evening meal for the family, who had been out at work and school all day. This was now my role. It gave me a purpose – I felt I was making a valuable contribution to the household – and at the same time ensured I got through the day without too much pain or exhaustion and at my own pace.

As time progressed I was able to contemplate adding further activities, such as a walk to the local shop, doing the vacuuming and so on. Things did not always go smoothly and plans had to be revised. My biggest concern was that I might meet someone in the street who wanted to stand and talk. Standing for only a couple of minutes left me so exhausted I would struggle to get home and the plans for the whole day would have to be abandoned. Even after almost 30 years I still have this problem so I find all sorts of diplomatic ways to avoid standing for whatever reason. Using walking aids such as sticks and crutches does not help. To have a conversation I need to sit down.

As you will have gathered, planning involves thinking seriously about how much you can manage to accomplish each day – in plain language, do not bite off more than you can chew! Make progress by taking small steps, one step at a time. You will be surprised how far you can travel in this way, and what is more you will feel the benefit of increasing energy.

Pace yourself through every activity. Break down every task into manageable chunks and tackle everything deliberately and in your own time. Go at your own pace and do not allow other people to impose their timetable on you. It is helpful to decide in advance how long you are going to spend on a task before having a break or finishing for the day. If it helps, set a timer and resolve to stop when it pings. When you take a break, make it at least half an hour, with time for a drink or to restore yourself with light exercise or a relaxation session. Once you start an activity do not get carried away by enthusiasm for the job. It will still be there when you are ready to come back to it.

Do not be your own worst enemy – a cautionary tale

Ron, a keen amateur artist with severely limited mobility and high blood pressure, had slowly recovered from a position where he was almost completely inactive, depressed and isolated to one where he was beginning to enjoy life once more. He had joined an art club and made new friends. He had shown his talent and skill as an artist in his schooldays but had not pursued his interest as he got older. As time went on Ron began to put more and more time and energy into his art work, competing for exhibition space in local shows and from time to time feeling the frustration of having his work rejected by selection panels.

However, as his art became more well known and admired he began to receive requests to show his work. Ron was asked to exhibit about a dozen paintings in his local community centre and to go along with his paintings at 2 p.m. the day before the exhibition was due to open. He arrived at the appointed time only to find the room was still being used by a mother and toddler group. When he eventually got into the room an hour later he was told he had to be finished by four o'clock as the room was booked for a committee meeting. In his anxiety to complete the hanging in time, he rushed with the measurements and the fixing. This was on top of working late into the previous night to complete the picture framing. The result was that instead of enjoying his success at the opening of the exhibition the following day, he was at home in bed, exhausted and racked with pain.

Over the years I have worked with many people who have devoted a great deal of time and energy, with the support of family, friends, colleagues and the expertise of professionals, to getting better. Free from the worst symptoms of their illness and feeling full of energy, sometimes buoyed up by their medication, they have abandoned the healthy lifestyle that brought about their healing and launched themselves into their old ways. They have worked to the point of exhaustion, competed for extra work, argued for a bigger margin, no matter how insignificant, on a business deal and have been unable to say no to any request for their services. Meals have been missed or rushed and exercise and relaxation have been felt to be no longer necessary. They have forgotten the basic rules of healing:

- Respect yourself in body, mind and spirit.
- Remember that this plan for healing depends on you following its prescription closely for the rest of your life.
- Remember that the changes you make need to be permanent.

It is easy to sabotage your achievements towards healing by back-sliding, but at this point I would like to draw your attention to the way your attempts at healing can be jeopardized even before you begin.

5

Get to know the inner you

If illness was entirely physical then healing would be very simple.

Chronic illness needs to be understood as part of a complex system of thoughts, feelings, emotions, attitudes and beliefs that are inextricably linked with the process of physical breakdown. The interaction of all of these elements is the result of a multitude of life experiences, some of which are good and strengthening, some of which are positively damaging. It is these life experiences that determine the way we view ourselves, the way we feel about life, the way we approach adversity and the way we conduct our relationships. You may have built up a belief that somehow you are not worthy of spending time and energy on your own well-being.

I have had many clients come to me for help who seemed unwilling to devote even half an hour to themselves each day, away from the family and their demands, in order to follow a relaxation programme. As a child you may have been taught to put others first, no matter how much it inconvenienced you. You probably all know the mother who struggles to get around while she is ill and in pain just so that she can be at the service of the rest of the family.

You may feel that your illness is the result of some transgression and is a punishment that you must bear with fortitude. It is common for people to search their memory in an effort to find some explanation for their illness, to find some proof that they have done wrong to someone and that their illness is a form of retribution. Anyone who carries a burden of guilt may find it difficult to enter wholeheartedly into a programme of self-management, and even if they do, they unconsciously find ways to sabotage any small improvements they might have made.

Think very carefully . . .

Do you doubt your own self-worth?

In other words, do you place a low value on yourself? It is so easy to develop feelings of inadequacy as we grow up, perhaps experiencing failures at school, being victims of bullying, subject to the excessive demands of parents, or perhaps even suffering physical or sexual abuse. You may develop feelings of inadequacy because you consider your job to be menial or think you have missed out in competition with others. Your self-image may be poor because you do not feel that you live up to ideals portrayed in the media. You may have a disability that makes you believe you are physically unattractive. Your self-esteem may be low following the breakdown of a relationship, or you may be caught in a relationship with a partner who constantly belittles you so that you no longer recognize your own good qualities. In my work I have come across partners who would prefer their wife or husband to remain ill and dependent on them for all decisions made in the home. I have experienced their aggression towards me for encouraging their partner to become more active and less isolated, even though improvements were clearly obvious.

Maureen had a painful form of arthritis that made walking difficult. She used two sticks and soon became exhausted so her husband took her everywhere by car. Her prolonged inactivity made her feel very unfit and she had put on a lot of weight. Maureen made good progress learning relaxation techniques, and during the course of our discussions she wondered whether her mobility might be improved by using her bicycle again. The idea worked: she felt liberated and was now able to venture out alone to local shops or to call on friends for a cup of tea and a gossip. Exhaustion was no longer a problem and she relished the feeling of having so much more energy. However, after a few weeks her husband stopped me in the street and objected strongly to my support of the idea of a bicycle. He reminded me that 'my wife is a sick woman!' He insisted that his wife terminate the treatment, and she reverted to her state of complete dependence and, eventually, experienced the onset of depression and resentment.

Some people appear to be born pessimists and it is difficult to shake their belief that nothing they or anyone else can do can improve their lot. This can be a real obstacle to getting better. It is important to get these people to make constant appraisal of all the good things that happen to them in the course of a day, a week and so on, and to recognize that more good things happen in life than bad. Focusing on the positive events in daily life gives a boost to anyone seeking to get better. Anticipating the worst and dwelling on the bad things that have happened to you in the past is no help at all.

We have to accept the evidence that psychological and emotional factors arising from life experiences play a great part in its causation so it is appropriate to take these factors into account in order to bring about healing. As a psychotherapist, my main task was to heal the person with the illness. As emotional healing took place and the person gained inner strength, the illness itself became less of a burden. My work often involved working with people to help them recognize how deeply buried feelings and emotions were making it difficult for them to cope with their illness or move on towards healing. The account of my own situation at the beginning of this book is an illustration of this.

Depression

An important part of discovering the 'inner you' involves learning more about the interaction between yourself and your illness. We have already discussed how the emotions triggered by the illness need to be recognized and dealt with before you can move on. Sometimes depression and anxiety are a normal response to the extraordinary situation brought about by the onset of chronic illness. If unrecognized or ignored, depression and anxiety can make your physical condition worse because they bring about bio-chemical changes that can hasten the progression of the disease, and as a result it becomes harder to take control of the illness.

In *The Pain Management Handbook* I draw attention to the problem of depression in relation to treating chronic pain. Sometimes pain is a symptom of depression and only careful testing and diagnosis can determine this. Treatment of the depression often sorts out a chronic pain problem. Depression can be a chronic illness in its own right and can often be overlooked. Half of people with depression remain undiagnosed, even though it is said to affect as many as one in five women and one in eight men in the UK at some time in their lives. Unfortunately, if people are not referred for a full pain assessment they may be treated inappropriately over a number of years for chronic pain rather than chronic depression, or vice versa. This is why it is so important to have a thorough medical and psychological investigation, not only with chronic pain but with any chronic illness where there appear to be symptoms of depression. Here are some of the symptoms you should be aware of, whether you have a chronic illness or not. They can make life really difficult:

- frequent bouts of crying and feeling sad
- difficulty sleeping or waking in the early hours unable to get back to sleep
- tiredness, exhaustion and irritability
- anxiety and feelings of agitation
- lack of concentration
- headaches
- loss of patience and overreacting
- making mountains out of molehills
- low sex drive, impotence
- general loss of interest in every aspect of life
- overdependence on medication
- feeling that everyone is against you.

Recognizing any of the symptoms in this list does not immediately indicate that you are suffering from depression, as anyone who has a long-term illness will testify. Many illnesses are debilitating and frightening and can bring on feelings of weakness, lassitude, inability to relate to others and a complete lack of interest in anything that is going on around you. You may even feel that your personality has changed completely. What is important is that you do not neglect these signs. Talk about them with your doctor and seek reassurance. If they persist, they will have a profound influence on your ability to cope with your illness. You may reach a stage where you feel helpless to influence your recovery or plan for the future.

The following case history is presented to illustrate how life experiences with strong emotional associations can influence the progression of an illness.

Jean's story

Jean's problems stemmed from an arthritic condition and so far she had not responded to medication and various forms of physical intervention. It was for this reason that, at the age of 55, she was referred to a pain management course. She had extremely sensitive feet that made it difficult for her to stand for any length of time and walking was painful and exhausting. Much of the time she used a wheelchair to get around, and on her feet she chose to wear very thick socks and slippers to cushion her soles and feet. Although she responded well to being part of the group and no longer felt so isolated, helpless and depressed, her feet still remained a problem. We had a case review involving Jean and the team together to try to find another way to help her.

The fact that she was being referred to me for psychotherapy treatment caused her concern as she thought that we must have concluded that she had some form of mental illness or that her pain was imagined. We explained that we all accepted that her pain was real and she was not being difficult, but that from time to time we had to make extra provision for anyone we felt was finding it difficult to make progress. She agreed to the plan out of desperation, feeling that all other avenues of help were now closed to her. I did not think she was confident that I could help her.

When we met it seemed that Jean wished to spend the time going over and over all of the negative aspects of her situation. It was difficult to get her to focus positively on the task in hand, that of exploring ways out of her problem. She felt her relationship with her husband was deteriorating as she was no longer a lively companion for him but merely a burden. Her social life had been completely destroyed and most household tasks left her exhausted and in pain.

She presented herself to me as a hard, bitter and controlling person caught up in a situation she was helpless to control, unable to see how anyone else could help her now that her medical treatment had proved unsuccessful. I must admit she seemed a tough nut to crack, but if healing was to happen I must meet the challenge.

Hypnosis would have been helpful but Jean would have none of it. This aversion to hypnosis is shared by many people in the population who fear being under the control of someone else. Popular fiction, films, TV and stage shows give a completely false portrayal of therapeutic hypnosis. People are used to seeing the hypnotist as taking over people's minds and making them do silly things for a laugh! Of course, the people involved may well have been 'planted' in the audience.

We agreed to try another approach. Jean was quite happy to continue 'our chats' as she maintained it was doing her good to 'get things off her chest'. This may have made her feel better temporarily, but constantly talking about the negative aspects of her life may have had the effect of reinforcing her bad feelings, and consequently her pain and isolation.

I explained that therapy is a two-way process and that it was important we move on from looking at the negative aspects of her present life. Although listening is part of the process of healing, something more is needed. I proposed that we continue by exploring the totality of her life: it would help me to get a fuller picture of her as a person and might throw some light on how her problem had developed. This joint exploration is important in psychotherapy as a basis for understanding the problem and for working out a treatment plan. However, the exploration itself can be effective in bringing about healing.

I was interested in her life history and Jean visibly relaxed as she talked, painting a picture of a reasonably happy childhood, schooling without pressure and no particular highlights or achievements, work in a neighbourhood clothing shop and, at 19, marriage to her husband, who worked as a joiner. In time they bought their own house and had two children who were now married with young families of their own. Her illness had started soon after her children had left home and her pain problem had progressively deteriorated.

The breakthrough came when I asked Jean about her interests and hobbies. She explained that she had always liked ballroom dancing – she had attended classes as a child, achieving all the various grades and taking part in competitions, and had married her dancing partner. She and her husband had only given up dancing when the children came along. I asked whether she had ever thought of taking it up again and she said that, in fact, she had. Soon after her elder son married she had started going to a ballroom dancing club once a week with her daughter-in-law, Linda. I remarked that her pain had probably put paid to that, at which point she became very quiet and then tears started to flow. She sobbed for a long time. It was some time before she recovered enough to explain that it was not her pain that made her give up dancing but the sudden death of her daughter-in-law as a result of an undiagnosed heart problem.

This turn of events was surprising but not uncommon when exploring someone's life history. Things we think buried suddenly spring from nowhere and have a very strong emotional impact. Feelings may be expressed which have been suppressed because of the need to put on a brave face for those around and because someone has to be strong and provide an anchor for others in the family. Very often the family unconsciously selects one member to be the strong one, to bear the burdens of the rest. You can often see this in the way parents and grandparents talk and relate to children as young as five or six who are expected to behave and carry responsibility way beyond their years, or to act as guardians to their younger siblings. In the same way families can select one of their members to 'carry the can' for everything that goes wrong – to be the scapegoat. That in its own way can be a heavy burden to carry and a child can consequently be limited in self-esteem.

The practical problems of helping her son and looking after his young child full-time had taken over Jean's life so she had not had the opportunity to grieve the loss of her daughter-in-law and good friend. She then began to talk about how important her relationship with Linda had been, saying they were like sisters and how much she missed her. It seemed that for the first time she was grieving appropriately rather than coping with practical matters. Her serious pain problem had set in after her son had found a new partner. She had not really approved of this, less than two years after her daughter-in-law's death, but she supposed it would work out for the best in the long run. Her amazed expression showed me that she had only that moment acknowledged how her pain was interwoven with her sense of loss. As she talked her voice softened, a new light appeared in her eyes, and the years seemed to drop away from her.

I saw Jean only once more after that session. She turned up without her wheelchair, wearing normal footwear. It was my turn to express amazement at her progress, but she explained that our last session had made her feel as though a burden had been lifted, so much so that in her excitement she had gone home and shared all that had happened in the session with her family. She was delighted when her husband suggested that a holiday would do them both good as he felt her true personality had returned. The pain and sensitivity was still there but it was manageable, and by pacing herself, practising relaxation and exercising she could get through the day without too much trouble. She thanked me for my help and said she thought she could cope quite well on her own from now on. Her parting gift to me was a brand new pair of thick-soled socks!

As you have seen from my own story and that of Jean, progress with healing may be blocked. In my case, strong feelings of anger relating to multiple losses I experienced following the onset of my illness were making my illness worse, and consequently my feelings of isolation were growing until Helen helped me to recognize and release them. Jean had not been able to grieve as she took on the task of being strong for her family. These two cases illustrate that we may need professional help in order to help us cope with the initial impact of chronic illness or to gain the emotional strength to continue coping or following a positive plan for healing.

The following case history illustrates once more that illnesses may need to be understood on an emotional level.

Barbara's story

Barbara came to see me seeking help. She was 45 years old and she was a successful businesswoman; she had never married. She explained that she had for many years suffered from digestive problems, hiatus hernia and inflammation of the bowel, and to ease the symptoms she used prescription and over-the-counter medicines. She put her problems down to stress as she worked virtually non-stop in her management consultancy business. She said she had come to see me at this time because in spite of her success she was getting no enjoyment from life. Her medical condition felt worse and she needed to feel better quickly as she had been invited to take part in a popular TV series.

This was a woman who drove herself hard and now, it seemed, she was making hard demands of me. I wondered why she should demand a quick fix from me when she had been under medical care for so many years. She said she had built up her business on the back of her own hard work and commitment and she made similar demands of her staff, who were well rewarded. She admitted that she seemed to be setting me an impossible task. I explained that she could not just hand over her problem to me as she had been used to doing with her GP. We would have to devise a way of working together, with probably more input from her than from me. I reminded her that she was a woman of undoubted intelligence and drive who invariably succeeded at whatever she took on and that together we would work towards releasing her own energy to use in bringing about her own healing.

Having cleared up that issue we agreed to a plan of action. I suggested that we could approach her problem two ways:

1 Under hypnosis I could teach her relaxation techniques and suggest ways she could ease the burden on herself.
2 Alternatively, I could explore with her the underlying reasons for her need to push herself so hard.

She thought that the idea of hypnosis was appealing and added that she would prefer to find the root of her problems.

We agreed that regression to earlier stages of her life might be helpful. In regression we explore different episodes of a person's life to see if he or she recognizes an event that has played a critical part in his or her development. Events which are particularly seen as important focus on experiences of loss, separation, trauma, physical or sexual assault, rape or other events which have a strong emotional content. For example, it may be something which at the time provokes extreme fear.

These events are significant in therapy because the person involved may have buried the very strong feelings experienced at the time, as a protective measure. Children, particularly when faced with a traumatic event, may not have the understanding or psychological and emotional maturity to come to terms with an experience which is terrifying. They may not be able to cope with being separated from a parent by death or understand that rows between warring parents are not the fault of the child. The strong feelings provoked are beyond the child's capacity to cope with at that time and as a safety measure are suppressed. The feelings may get buried deep in the unconscious, where they fester, producing physical, psychological or emotional problems at a later date. They may be instrumental in producing an illness or preventing healing from taking place.

As a therapist it is the feeling content accompanying the episode that I try to unlock. This mechanism is not exclusive to children; adults can be overwhelmed at any time, hence the need for people to be supported at times of extreme or continued stress. Recognition of the problems that can arise for people experiencing stressful events has led to the development of therapies for managing what is now termed post-traumatic stress syndrome.

The regression revealed nothing remarkable in Barbara's life until we reached her final year in university. At that point she became very quiet and it was clear to see in her face and posture that she was troubled and experiencing strong emotions. I allowed her a few minutes before asking what she was experiencing. She saw herself in childbirth, and when it was over saw and felt the child, a boy she was told, being taken away to be placed for adoption. She never saw the child again. All she was left with was a feeling of emptiness. Within days she was back at university where she threw herself into her studies, working so hard day and night that she achieved a first class honours degree.

We talked for a long time about her 'forgotten pregnancy' and the unacknowledged feelings of shame and fear. We talked about the agonizing decision she had made to part with the baby. She had not told her parents of the pregnancy, which she kept secret from all but a few. She had avoided going home during that time, claiming the need to work and go on field trips. At that time getting her degree was all that seemed to matter. We spent most of our time talking about her feelings at giving up the baby. For the first time ever she talked about her guilt and shame and how awful she felt inside – like having a stone weighing her down. She had been desperate to hold the baby and for someone to hold her, but the baby had been taken away – and there was no one there for her.

Following the cathartic but nevertheless healing experience of the regression, she was able to focus on devising a plan to get more balance between work and other aspects of her life and finding helpful ways to reduce the stress surrounding her digestive problems. The plan involved working with me for a couple of sessions to learn the skills of deep relaxation. We discussed in these sessions how she might devote her newfound energy to planning a more suitable diet, allowing time for meals and following new avenues other than those involving work. She realized that it was not really necessary to devote every waking hour to her company; she had only been trying to fill the void in her life by doing something worthy.

Emotion and healing

Both these cases illustrate how very strong emotional experiences can interfere with the healing process, and may in fact have a lot to do with the onset of an illness. Neither of these ladies would have made any progress without psychotherapy. Once the emotional obstacles at the root of their problems had been recognized, they were able to move on to making plans that meant looking at all aspects of their lives – diet, relationships, work, leisure, exercise and means of coping with stress.

6

Work on your confidence and self-esteem

It may be that your illness has shattered your confidence and lowered your self-esteem to such an extent that you have found it increasingly difficult to communicate with others, make decisions or assert yourself in a way that is acceptable to those around you. We have already looked at the way in which your attitudes and emotional responses may hinder your attempts to get on with others or to make positive changes. Many of your attitudes and emotional responses may not result directly from your present problems; for many years you may have harboured some inner discomfort which adds to your tension and you may not be in full control of your life. I want to try to help you to identify the source of this discomfort. It may be that other people, hangovers from the past, your previous learning, or attitudes and beliefs passed on to you when you were a child have had a profound influence on the way you are coping now. Any of these can lower your self-esteem, be a major source of stress and hinder your attempts at self-management.

I have prepared a list of statements which may or may not apply to you. Study them, think about them and see how many are relevant. Some will apply to all of us, but if you find yourself agreeing with most of them then it is time to make changes for your own benefit. It is important to acknowledge which aspects of living are contributing to your distress, and to sort out what it is that is limiting your ability to help yourself.

- I believe there may be something basically wrong with me that is making me unhappy.
- I feel guilty when I am having my own way, even over something trivial.
- I don't like to 'rock the boat' even when something does not seem right.
- I feel guilty when I shirk a domestic duty – neglect to clean the

house, leave the washing up overnight, do not have meals ready on time.

- I feel uneasy if my partner does not have a meal ready for me when I come home.
- I think I should be able to cope with any situation and that it is a sign of failure to ask for help.
- I believe that in politics, business and science, men are naturally smarter.
- An inner voice tells me that it is the job of a 'good woman' always to look after her man.
- I believe I am not allowed to show anger. I feel angry about my situation but feel I cannot talk about it.
- I feel guilty about spending money on myself unless I have someone else's approval.
- I still seek the approval, not just the advice, of my parents for major decisions in my life.
- I find it hard to accept compliments. I often think they are insincere.
- I would do almost anything to avoid an argument or confrontation.
- My mother or father comes to mind when I 'disobey' a rule that I was taught as a child, and I expect to be punished.
- I believe that all rules need to be followed because they are made by people whose judgement is better than mine.
- I accept invitations to do things with friends or family even when I would rather not and then resent them for aggravating my pain or discomfort.
- If I am enjoying myself I expect discomfort to follow automatically, so I turn down opportunities to go out.
- I am afraid to try anything new in case I fail and make a fool of myself.
- I resist new experiences and have not done anything different for more than a month.
- I feel guilty and uneasy if I am away from home for too long and I feel upset when something disrupts my daily routine.
- I feel that others do not believe that my illness is as bad as I make out and I find myself talking about it frequently, to convince them.
- I tackle DIY jobs because I think it is expected of me even although I know I am not up to it.
- I truly feel that sacrificing myself for others makes me a better person even if it means ignoring my own needs.

- I jump up immediately to answer the doorbell or telephone. I drop everything to respond to an immediate demand.
- I am staying in a bad relationship because I would not know where to turn if I were alone.
- I am afraid to make positive steps to improve my condition because I feel I will lose out in other ways.

If a substantial number of these statements apply to you then you have some serious thinking to do, as they will help to highlight the areas you need to work on. In my experience, just becoming aware of where you stand is enough to start a process of change and self-improvement.

I am not suggesting that there is a simple solution to every problem or that it is easy to make the necessary changes. However, it is most important to question those areas of life which are causing distress, to ask yourself, 'Is this how I want to live?' and then to have the courage to work towards change. You may need some help to assert yourself and overcome your fear of upsetting other people, especially those close to you who may be quite unaware of the way you feel.

Self-esteem is the value you put on yourself. People who suffer from long-term illness or chronic disability are in danger of losing their self-esteem and confidence. This loss of self-esteem follows the loss of physical ability. It is made worse by knock-on effects such as losing a job and being unable to provide for the family financially and physically, becoming dependent on the state or placing the burden of financial security on a partner. Self-esteem plummets even further if the illness makes a person feel he or she is no longer sexually attractive and is 'past it'.

When you get setbacks, old problems resurface and your attempts to rebuild your life are threatened as you face once again the possibility of loss. The threat exposes you once more to the negative feelings of anger and rage that were a part of your grief when you first had to face up to the fact that your illness had taken away so many parts of your life experience. At this point some people feel they are so worthless they might as well give up and not even try do those things that they know can help them. Many people make a start at rebuilding their lives, but because their negative feelings have not been dealt with and laid to rest they can find themselves sabotaging their own efforts. It is no fault of theirs but a sign that they need professional help to grieve and lay their ghosts.

Talking about your feelings is important and will help to remove much of the confusion and negativity that can so easily dominate your mind. No one is exempt from feelings of worthlessness. They recur from time to time with everybody, whether you have an illness or not, but if you recognize that these powerful emotions are an obstacle to your progress then talk to your doctor about them. Your doctor can arrange for you to have psychological help through the NHS if he or she feels this is appropriate. It may be that this service is not generally available in your area because resources are limited. However, try to avoid seeking refuge in tranquillizers or alcohol; these will not help to solve your situation. If you are religious, do not underestimate the role of your local clergy, who are trained in pastoral care and are more than willing to listen, guide and restore in times of personal crisis.

Avoiding conflict can be a sign of strength

It is important to recognize that when you have an illness that has reduced your physical capacity, weakened your spirit and reduced your confidence and self-esteem, you are very vulnerable. Your ability to meet challenges of any sort is limited. Remember that an injured lion will soon lose his status as leader of the pride as stronger beasts seize their opportunity to depose him. I know from experience that it is wiser to step back from potential conflict, because I feel that my energy would be wasted and I know that I would emerge with my confidence and self-esteem, which have been rebuilt after many years, badly dented. The feeling of physical and emotional bruising remains for a long time after the event. This is in complete contrast to the way I was before my illness, when I would launch myself into any challenge confronting me. As soon as the matter was cleared up I was ready to move on to the next. Now I have to keep reminding myself daily of the things I have set my mind on achieving and to tell myself that any negative feelings will pass and that the energy will return, knowing that the coping skills I have learned, and which I am passing on to you, will see me through.

It is time now to think about recognizing and rebuilding your own self-worth and to get in touch with the real person inside. In our society much value is placed on being able to work. If you cannot work you feel in some way diminished. In my own case, even though my chosen career was ended, I had to find ways of satisfying myself I was a useful citizen and re-trained for a job I could do part-time from home. It was not until I reached retirement age that the feeling I owed it to someone to be working became less of a pressure.

So how do you tackle your own rehabilitation?

- When you have finished this book, set aside at least 30 minutes each day for exercise and set aside the same amount of time at least twice a day for a relaxation session.
- Practise diaphragmatic breathing at every opportunity until it is second nature (see Chapter 7).
- Simplify your life as much as possible (see page 92 on exercise and relaxation).
- Set your own agenda. Do not try to keep up with others, especially if they are half your age.
- Know your own limitations and do not be afraid to tell people what they are. You cannot expect others to be mind readers.
- Share your worries with people close to you and work with them to sort out any problems – for example, financial, legal, medical, social. If you keep them to yourself they can easily get out of proportion.
- Stand tall.
- Find confident and positive people to be with.
- Keep visualizing times when you felt most confident.
- Do not give yourself a hard time.
- If you talk yourself down, then you will feel down. Say over and over again, 'I'm a great person, I'm getting better each day and my best is yet to come.'

Progress in your rehabilitation may not be easy and will take time, but the more you put in, the more you get out!

As your friends and family see the change they will respond differently to you and find their own ways of rewarding you to show how much they value and appreciate you. They may have been doing this all along, but because you have been weighed down by your feelings of loss, confusion and anger you have not been able to see it.

Whatever you feel you are achieving as you make progress, remember that your self-esteem needs to be worked on throughout life. You may not be able to work full-time as you used to, or bring in a salary, and you may not hold an important position because of your illness, but everybody reaches this stage at some time and this may be one of the reasons for decline in old age. People start to feel they need not bother to keep up appearances. Then it is 'I can't be bothered to have my hair cut or set and I have enough clothes to "see me through"' . . . 'I have lost a few teeth but I don't want to spend money on dentists at my age' and so on. Thus begins the downward spiral which leads to the grumpy old man and woman syndrome. People with chronic illness can so easily, at any age, portray this negative image associated with some old people. It is so much easier to sit with feet up, nibbling on chocolate biscuits while you watch daytime TV. This is not you, though, is it?

To increase your confidence and self-esteem further, make a list of ten positive statements about yourself. Keep reminding yourself frequently of these positive affirmations. These represent the real you. You may find this difficult at first and you may need to think about it. You may even need prompting from those close to you. What is important is that you list those things that *you* think are positive qualities. Don't be modest but do be honest. We all have good qualities. Other people may see your good qualities but if you have lost sight of them it is time to give yourself a reminder. Make your list, pin it up somewhere you can see it and look at it frequently. Why not hang it near a mirror, then you can check yourself out, noting your posture and the care you have taken with your appearance.

More importantly, you can practise your smiling routine. This is a very simple and effective means of setting yourself up for the day: just go to a mirror as soon as you get up and give yourself a big smile! At the same time, remind yourself that you are really going to enjoy the day ahead. It helps to smile at as many people as you can, at every opportunity. In this way you train your face to appear to others as a smiley face whether you are consciously smiling or not, and you will be surprised how many people respond to you. It is a very healing experience. Smiling does much to cultivate a positive attitude, which the American Psychological Association reports has as big an impact on your life as giving up smoking or taking regular exercise. Do not limit your smile to the privacy of home. Take it with you when you go out!

Set yourself targets to achieve each week. Make them manageable. Tell people what you intend to do and accept their encouragement. With each success your confidence will grow. Do not forget to reward your success with a treat. Do not forget that whenever you achieve or make a change you move to a new place and from there you have a new perspective – you see things differently. You start the next challenge from a new place!

With each successive change your personality, which may have been masked for a long time, will begin to shine through and your feeling of 'self' will become stronger.

Your plan for healing
PART 2

Creating energy

Stress is what we feel normally when we are faced with a threat or a challenge. It is vital to our survival. It sets in motion a chain of physiological reactions in the body resulting in chemicals being released, such as adrenalin that gives us a sudden surge of energy to help us cope. You have probably heard stories of mothers who, finding their child in danger, have been able to perform enormous feats of strength such as lifting a car to release the child trapped beneath it. When the danger is past the body returns to its normal state. If the stress continues for any length of time, the adrenalin becomes depleted, energy is exhausted and the body is likely to suffer damage.

Coping with any illness, whether it be acute or chronic, requires energy. The stress that accompanies the illness can consume even more energy than the illness itself and result in creating further symptoms. Stress seems to accompany many chronic illnesses. Any disturbance that throws the body or mind out of balance produces the emotions of fear, anxiety, anger, disappointment, guilt and maybe even shame. If the illness continues indefinitely then there is every likelihood that the stress will also continue, resulting in fatigue, depression and low spirits, all signs that adrenalin and energy have been depleted. At this point the immune system is weakened and further health problems may be added, such as digestive difficulties, inflammatory illnesses, allergies, disturbed sleep and depression. We have to find ways of dealing with the stress and creating energy.

When we have pain or our illness seems to be getting worse we can feel overwhelmed. It seems there is no way we can control what is happening to us and we feel helpless. This is very destructive. We are shaken to the core and we get anxious. We may even go into a downward spiral, and when we reach the bottom it is a dark lonely place from which there seems to be no way back. Regaining control of our lives when we seem to have lost it completely may seem impossible. Having control over our lives involves exercising our ability to make choices. When we feel helpless there seems to be little scope for us to make *any* choices which will improve our condition. Despite this there is something we can do: it might seem a small and insignificant action, but we can choose to change the way we breathe. A small change indeed, but one which can lead to many bigger changes.

7

Breathing is the key to getting back in control

Poor breathing is a factor in asthma, high blood pressure, sleep disorders, stress, anxiety, headaches, all painful conditions, allergies, lack of energy, MS and ME. Good breating can alleviate unpleasant symptoms arising from other illnesses such as psoriasis and eczema. Breathing is the best-kept secret for improving your health.

Breathing is one of those functions that is partly under conscious control but for the most part continues without us thinking about it. If we can bring our breathing under control and it feels good, what is to say we cannot take control of other bodily functions? Evidence and personal experience show that we can control our breathing and achieve a state of relaxation, change our heart rate, reduce blood pressure – and lower pain levels.

These unconscious processes are directly influenced by the way we breathe. We just need to learn how. Once you have learned this method you will find it helps to control your pain, reduce anxiety, ease depression, improve sleep, lower blood pressure, help your body eliminate impurities and reduce the impact of your symptoms. In fact, every aspect of your health will benefit.

- When we are anxious or tense we breathe in a shallow way, high in the chest, increasing tension in all parts of the body.
- Babies breathe correctly, completely relaxed and with the breath moving in and out of the diaphragm or tummy area. As we grow older we tend to lose this rhythmic, relaxing way of breathing. We experience fear, anxiety. We become tense and the rhythm is upset.
- Incorrect breathing creates tense muscles and reduces the oxygen supply to the rest of the body. This produces a vicious circle of tension, leading to anxiety and fear, leading to more tension, leading to increased anxiety and fear . . . People with tension often have a disturbed sleep pattern resulting in fatigue and low

energy levels. If you add chronic pain to this vicious circle then the illness becomes so much more serious and more difficult to handle. Exhausted, tense bodies are strong candidates for more pain and anxiety. Streams of negative thoughts and images will attack the mind. The quickest way to release this tension is to re-learn how to breathe properly and develop ways of blocking out negativity.

- Correct diaphragmatic breathing helps break this vicious circle by releasing tension. Many people who learn this technique have told me how effective it is as a therapeutic aid, and for them it has been enough to help them live full lives without the need for medication.
- Initially you will need to set aside times to practise the breathing technique. Eventually it will become second nature, automatic and unconscious. You will recognize those situations which upset your breathing rhythm and work towards regaining your composure through breathing. Remember, breathing is the basis of life so it is important that we do it right. Apart from pain episodes, the most common life events which upset breathing are arguments, times when you are kept waiting on the telephone while the operator at the other end goes through a list of options, moments when you feel your computer has a life of its own and you are ready to throw it through the window, occasions when your children test your patience . . . You will no doubt be able to add a few more.

Diaphragmatic breathing

Diaphragmatic breathing is a skill you once had but have forgotten over your lifetime. I will show you how to regain this skill, which is at the heart of meditation programmes, hypnotherapy, yoga, t'ai chi and the martial arts. Once you have mastered this technique you will be able to use it whenever you want, and with practice it will become second nature and you will not have to think about it.

Learn to monitor your breathing throughout the day. The rhythm of your breathing changes according to whatever you are doing, and from time to time you may find that your breathing is high in your chest and there is tightness in your chest and shoulders. These changes happen unconsciously – when you are talking, thinking, driving, worrying, watching an exciting TV programme, listening to someone else's tale of woe, or when you are emotionally or sexually aroused. When you are aware of situations that affect your breathing then it will be possible to take note of any changes instantly and correct your breathing pattern. As your skill develops you will notice improvements in the way you feel, the way you relate to other people and the way you cope with stressful situations. The increased oxygen in your blood will make you feel brighter and more energetic and other people will notice the changes – maybe even before you do! I remember people remarking to me shortly after I started the pain management programme how my face had changed. I no longer looked so haggard. The only thing that had changed was my breathing pattern.

If you are beginning to relax after long periods of tension or anxiety it is quite possible that your mind will focus on anxious thoughts and feelings of anger and resentment about your situation or other people. Later on I will deal more fully with this topic (see Chapter 9), but for the time being remember this is your quiet time and just let any thoughts that come into your mind drift through. Don't hold on to them. Let them go. They are not important.

It is very easy to learn powerful techniques for healing and it need not cost you a penny!

When people come to me with a health or personal problem it is my practice to take a case history. This gives me an opportunity to listen and to observe body language, posture, facial expressions and, in particular, the way they breathe. The next step is to teach a series of breathing techniques that help induce a relaxed state and establish a good foundation for healing. When we are distressed, anxious or in pain our breathing is usually high in the chest, and muscles in that area, in the shoulders and in the abdomen are tense. As a result oxygen does not easily get into the bloodstream and reach the brain and numerous muscles and nerve cells in our body. Learning to breathe properly brings many benefits resulting from improved blood flow, increased relaxation, more efficient functioning of the organs of the body and elimination of waste and toxins.

It bears repeating that breathing is an automatic process that goes on without us thinking about it; we are usually unaware that it is happening beyond our control. However, we can learn to control our breathing, and as we do so we learn that other things happening outside our conscious awareness can also be controlled. As we develop our breathing skills we may find that tense muscles become relaxed, pain disappears or improves, we sleep better, our blood pressure reduces, our digestion improves, and our movement becomes more fluid. We may even find that the way we think, feel and behave changes for the better.

The technique I am going to demonstrate can be learned straight from these pages. You need no one else to read it for you, neither do you need the material to be recorded. Simply follow the instructions, and by the time you have read the passage you will be well on the way to learning a skill which is at the basis of self-healing. There is growing scientific evidence that relaxation, meditation, self-hypnosis and biofeedback can improve many medical and psychological conditions.

The aim of this simple technique is to help you to detach your mind and to quieten any negative thoughts. The intrusive running commentary that goes on in your mind much of the time without you realizing it takes a great deal of energy that you can ill afford. This negative activity is wasteful of energy when you have to cope with everyday life. In easing your mind and your body sufficiently to allow healing to take place, this technique is the first stage in relieving you of stress and allowing you to experience being in control of things going on in your body.

Step 1: Observe your breathing

Uncross your legs and place your feet flat on the floor. Now just breathe in and out slowly through the nose without effort. Breathe normally: do not attempt to change your breathing pattern. Observe the passage of air as you breathe in and out. Focus all your attention on your breathing. Put the book aside for a moment and sit for a few minutes breathing in this way.

How was that? Did you find that thoughts intruded as you carried out this exercise? If they did, do not worry. It is very difficult to block thoughts coming into your mind. When they do, just note that they are there and let them go . . . Now, repeat the exercise for a few minutes with full awareness focused on your breathing. You may find that it is almost impossible to detect the point at which your in breath becomes your out breath.

Step 2: Relaxation through breathing

Now that you have completed the first part of the exercise you can move on and lay the foundation for a form of breathing that will help you stay calm and relaxed in whatever situation you happen to find yourself. It is a technique that is at the heart of the therapeutic work of hypnosis, meditation and other forms of deep relaxation.

This time, as you read, breathe in for a count of five and, without holding your breath, breathe out through the nose to a count of five. Try not to pause between the in breath and the out breath. Make the operation as seamless as possible. As you continue, make your breathing slower and deeper. Always direct your breathing to a point halfway between your navel and your ribs, i.e. into your diaphragm. You will feel your diaphragm rise and fall with the breath. The more you practise, the more this will become your normal way to breathe. Continue to breathe in this way for a few minutes as you become aware of your own breathing rhythm. If you find this difficult or if you catch your breath, do not worry: you will soon develop a smooth rhythm which will help you to relax.

I am now going to ask you to pause in your reading as you focus completely on your breathing for the next five minutes, before we carry on to the next stage. Remember – let go of any obtrusive thoughts. If you wish, you may close your eyes.

How did you find that?

Breathing in this way needs practise. To practise effectively you need to set aside time for yourself in a quiet place away from any intrusions such as the telephone or members of the family. If you question your ability to do this then you also have to question just how committed you are to self-healing. Setting aside time and space for yourself is a good demonstration of your self-worth. When I was learning this skill I initially found I had to withdraw from the family situation to a room on my own for half an hour or so. I explained to the children that this was my 'homework' time and I was not to be disturbed. They soon accepted it and it was amusing to overhear one of them answering the phone in the hall saying, 'Daddy is unavailable, he's doing his homework.' One of my hypnotherapy clients who worked in a very busy office found refuge in his car every lunchtime.

The aim is to become mindful of your breathing wherever you are or whatever you are doing. It is so easy, under stress, for your breathing to become laboured, for your chest and throat to become tight and for tension to build up in muscles throughout the body restricting blood flow, restricting the capacity of organs to function well and in turn making the body a target for illness or making an existing problem worse. Take note of the way you breathe

- when you are holding on the phone, waiting for a call centre to answer or go through their list of options;

- when you are sitting in your car at traffic lights;
- when you are waiting for your favourite football team to score;
- when you are waiting for an exam result;
- when you are in the dentist's waiting room;
- when you cannot get off to sleep.

You can no doubt think of many more potentially stressful situations. Out of curiosity, what is your breathing like at this moment? Remember the breathing pattern – five in and five out! Re-establish this breathing pattern and keep it going. This is just the start but it is a crucial step as you begin the healing process. Many people I work with who have chronic pain report that just by adopting this simple breathing pattern they can actually bring their pain under control, and I agree because I practise it to control my own ever-present pain so that it rarely overwhelms me.

Even if you do nothing else for the rest of the day, master this breathing technique. Take every opportunity today and every day to sit quietly and allow this breathing rhythm to develop. It may be the first time you have shown respect for your body and your mind. It may be the first time you have not allowed other people or persistently ringing phones to dictate your thoughts and actions. The reaction of most people reading this would be: 'But this is impossible. So many people depend on me, want my advice, make demands. I have to meet deadlines, cook meals, meet children out of school . . .' the list goes on. I know all too well. Fit people can become sick people by trying to be 'all things to all men'. People who already have chronic illness risk becoming completely incapacitated and useless to themselves and anyone else if they fail to accept their limitations and the need for 'me' time.

This breathing technique, and allocating time for it, is fundamental for your survival. I have discussed this point more times than I can remember with groups I have been working with and have met resistance to bringing about the changes necessary. Oh yes, we all want to feel better – but not if it means adjusting our timetables. Much easier if we can take a pill and wait for everything to sort itself out. But beware: if you are not prepared to put aside the time to devote to your well-being, you are in fact contributing to your condition. How's your breathing now? Five in and five out!

I had a landlady once when I was on a fellowship in London. She was a very busy practice nurse in a poor London borough. She was subjected to many physical and emotional demands from her patients and their families and was convinced that the only way she could survive was by making time for meditation, so she got up early every morning to prepare her mind and body for the demands of the day. When she came home in the evening she went straight to her room for half an hour's meditation to clear her mind of the clutter built up during the day.

I will not say any more to convince you to put aside periods during the day for your own benefit. What is important at this stage is that you learn how to breathe consciously in the five-in-and-five-out rhythm until it becomes habit and you breathe in this way without having to think about it. Until now your breathing may have been outside your conscious awareness, but whenever you have been subject to various stresses your breathing has changed – usually for the worse, so that your brain, nerves and muscles have not received enough oxygen, your blood flow has been restricted and symptoms from your illness have been emphasized.

8

Progressive Muscle Relaxation

Recognizing tension and relaxation

It is important to develop an awareness of when you are tense and when you are relaxed. At times you may think you are relaxed but your muscles can still be holding on to tension. Many people think relaxation means lounging on the sofa watching TV or sitting over a pint in the pub. This is not the case!

Progressive Muscle Relaxation helps you to reduce the *resting tension* in your muscles by tensing and then relaxing individual muscle groups in various parts of the body. As a result you become increasingly aware of areas that may be holding tension and with practise you will be able to distinguish between states of tension and relaxation. Once you have reached that stage you are well on the way to controlling your pain, reducing agitation, getting rid of anxiety states or preventing undesirable symptoms from gaining ascendancy. The technique has been shown to be successful in treating and preventing stress-related conditions such as high blood pressure, tension headaches and pain. In my own work with clients I have used it successfully in treating people with anxiety states as well as painful conditions. It was developed early in the twentieth century by Edward Jacobson, a US physiologist, who maintained that anxiety resulted in muscle tension and that reducing this tension would allow the body's stress response to diminish.

When we have pain we tend to tense other parts of our body to compensate. This tension can become a permanent feature of our lives if we allow it to, and as a result many people experience generalized pain that does not seem to be focused in one particular spot, with the whole body sore and subject to spasm. I often talk to people I am working with about the importance of 'putting the pain back in its rightful place'. In the same way it is important to put any symptoms of chronic illness in their place – as just a part of you and your daily life, not the dominant feature. It is so easy for a medical problem to take over your life to the exclusion of all else. For example, you might start off with back pain and over time experience pain throughout your body. When this happens you can feel as though your condition has deteriorated or that you have developed cancer or some other potentially fatal condition. We fear the worst as our anxiety grows. The result may be more visits to the doctor, increasing medication, becoming more isolated, anxious and depressed. It does not have to be like this!

Learning the skill of Progressive Muscle Relaxation can directly help us to relieve the body of its disabling tensions. A study in 2004 in the Purdue School of Nursing in Indiana showed that Progressive Muscle Relaxation achieved significant reductions in pain and mobility problems for osteoarthritis patients. A big advantage of practising Progressive Muscle Relaxation is that it can be carried out anywhere without the need for any special equipment. All you need to do is to sit or lie down in a comfortable position and focus on the various muscle groups in turn.

It is such a powerful method of relaxation that you may find it is the only skill you need to help you cope with your pain and anxieties. No matter how many setbacks you have, it will work every time. For some people it is as though they are experiencing full and deep relaxation for the first time.

As an aid I have recorded the following Progressive Muscle Relaxation sequence on CD as a relaxation programme and this can be ordered for a nominal charge from Pain Association Scotland, who benefit from the sale of this and other CDs that I have recorded. Details are given at the end of the book (see Useful addresses).

Instructions for Progressive Muscle Relaxation

1 Sit in a fully supported position on a chair or lie down on your back on the floor. If lying down, cover yourself with a blanket or duvet. Become aware of your breathing for a minute or two. Experience the in breath flowing into the diaphragm and allow your out breath to flow easily and comfortably, without any pause between the in and out breaths. When your breathing is steady and comfortable, focus your attention on your arms. Lift them slightly, extend them and clench your fists as hard as you can; hold your breath to a count of five. Let the tension go, breathing out as you do so, and let the arms fall back into the resting position. Repeat this exercise three times. Take note of the way your

muscles feel now that they are relaxed. Feel the warmth of the increased blood flow into your arms, hands and fingers.

2 Take a deep breath and hold it; at the same time, raise your shoulders towards your ears, pulling your head down towards your shoulders. Hold the breath and the tension for a count of five, then release the breath and the tension and allow the shoulders to relax completely. Repeat three times.

3 Take a deep breath into the chest and hold it for a count of five while tensing the muscles in the chest area, then let go of the breath and the tension, allowing all the muscles to relax completely. Repeat three times.

Take a moment to rest and breathe comfortably into your diaphragm for several moments. Now, in your own time, carry on with the next step.

4 If you are lying down, bend your knees slightly. Now tighten the muscles around your abdomen and pelvic area. Breathe in, hold the breath and the tension for a count of five, then let go the breath and the tension. Repeat three times.

This is a good point to pause and take note of what is happening in your body. You should be aware of an increased blood flow and a feeling of warmth beginning to spread through your body. Check your breathing again. Is it calm and steady? As you continue with these exercises, make sure you breathe out completely as you let go the tension.

5 Tighten the muscles of your buttocks as hard as you can. Take a deep breath and hold the tension and the breath for a count of five. Let go the tension and the breath, allowing the muscles to relax completely. Repeat three times.

6 Tighten the muscles of the thighs as hard as you can. Take a deep breath and hold the tension and the breath for a count of five. Let go the tension and the breath, letting the muscles relax completely. Repeat three times.

7 With your feet together and legs stretched out in front of you, tighten the muscles of your feet and calves by pointing your toes *away* from you as hard as you can. Take a deep breath and hold the tension and the breath for a count of five. Now, let go the tension and the breath, allowing the muscles to relax completely. Repeat three times.

8 With feet together and legs stretched out in front of you, tighten the muscles of your feet and calves by pointing your toes *towards* you as far as you can. Take a deep breath and hold the tension and the breath for a count of five. Now, let go the tension and the breath, allowing the muscles to relax completely. Repeat three times.

Now, rest quietly for a few moments. Restore your breathing into your diaphragm and experience the feeling of complete relaxation throughout your whole body.

9 This final exercise is particularly good for people with head, face and neck pains. Try not to be self-conscious about this one. Set out to enjoy it. If you feel like laughing, go ahead, because laughter helps to reduce tension better than any other exercise! Start by tightening the muscles around the jaw and neck area. At the same time stretch the mouth into a grinning expression, stick out your tongue as far as you can, screw up your eyes, take a deep breath, hold the tension and count to five. Then let go the tension and the breath and relax completely. Repeat three times.

9

Calming your mind

Although you will soon find many benefits from the breathing exercises and progressive muscle relaxation, you can derive still more benefit by building a range of mental activities into your breathing exercises which will help calm your mind, clear away obtrusive unbidden thoughts and, even more importantly, stimulate beneficial hormones that will help you to change the way you feel, the way you behave, the way you relate to other people. Believe me, these changes will help you to cope with the unpleasant symptoms of your illness and, as many people find, they can do much to relieve the symptoms altogether. Most importantly, you will find that you are in control of what is happening in your body – and in your mind. This is your eureka moment!

Many people with chronic illness complain that as soon as they lie down to rest they are bombarded with a constant stream of disturbing, negative thoughts that destroys any prospect of sleep and increases fatigue and stress. As you gain control of your thoughts these problems should disappear.

To help you, I would like you to try the following exercise as you continue to breathe slowly and deeply. This is a very simple exercise that will enable you to calm your mind, shutting off the internal dialogue. Although it is simple, it is an exercise that can have profound effects on your physiology. As you continue the exercise you will stimulate the relaxation reflex when beneficial hormones are released in your brain, having a direct influence on any feelings of depression, anxiety and pain. These hormones can help lower blood pressure, improve drainage from the lymphatic system and ultimately induce a greater sense of well-being.

Here is a new breathing rhythm. Breathe in to a count of four, hold your breath for a count of four and exhale for a count of six. So establish this new rhythm and for the next few minutes, as your relaxation deepens, with each out breath express the word 'calm' or 'uumm . . .' (the accepted sound used in meditation practice). Hold the 'mm' as a humming sound as long as you can, either silently or aloud. As your skill develops you will find that it is possible to reach a depth of relaxation where it seems you are neither asleep nor fully awake – a comfortable drifting state. Do not read any further for the next few minutes, just do the exercise and enjoy the experience.

So, how did that feel? Remember, you can do this exercise at any time during a busy day, when preparing for sleep or getting back to sleep if you have been disturbed. It is an exercise I have taught to people wishing to learn self-hypnosis. It is also an exercise that, as the basis of meditation, involves closing the mind to outside distractions, developing relaxation and quieting of the mind even in noisy or crowded places.

The healing power of music

Do not underestimate the power of music to induce calmness and relaxation or to invigorate. Make a point of listening to music every day, perhaps when you are practising relaxation or meditating. The ideal music for this has about 60 beats per minute, in time with the resting heartbeat. Our bodies automatically adjust to the pace, rhythm and pulse of the music. Sitting silently, breathing slowly and deeply, increases our ability to listen, and when this happens the music penetrates the whole of our body and the sound can then work on healing, increasing our well-being. Research indicates that music has the effect of improving respiration, lowering blood pressure, increasing blood flow, relaxing muscle tension and reducing anxiety. People also report significant reduction in pain levels. I can support this view as I have used music therapeutically with patients for almost 30 years. The slow movements of symphonies are ideal. The following are good examples of music for relaxation:

- Mozart Piano Concerto No. 21, slow movement.
- Stuart Mitchell, Suite for Orchestra.
- The slow movements of any Vivaldi symphony.
- Try listening to *Smooth Classics at Ten* on Classic FM. It is a good preparation for sleep.
- The piece of music that, in my opinion, has the greatest potential for healing is *The Lark Ascending* by Vaughan Williams.

Music, apart from relaxing, can also invigorate, create energy and reduce depression. Take time each day to listen to some up-beat music; what you choose depends on your taste, but you could try Tom Jones, Bobby Darin, Robbie Williams or Latin-American dance rhythms. Move around to the music – sing or hum along.

Music also has the power to evoke memories. When you hear a piece of familiar music it brings back memories, and your body at once responds with chemical changes that increase well-being.

10

Meditation

Meditation can help people develop their concentration, alertness, mental efficiency and creativity. Those who practise meditation benefit from lowered blood pressure, reductions in heart and breathing rates, lowered anxiety and greater tolerance of stress, and there is evidence that the stress hormones such as epinephrine and cortisone are reduced. The hormone melatonin, which regulates sleep, is increased through meditation. Research also suggests that meditation has beneficial effects on the immune system, which helps increase the ability to resist illness and to heal existing conditions. Meditation is often referred to as Mindful Meditation. It can be practised throughout life.

In my research for this book I interviewed Rosanne, who I knew would have some interesting things to say on the subject of breathing and meditation and their value for helping people with chronic illness.

About 20 years ago, Rosanne had to give up work owing to repetitive strain injury and stress. She had relentless pain, sleepless nights and fatigue that went with the pain and lack of sleep. She was desperate. By chance she saw a notice advertising a yoga class. She joined and in the following weeks gained much benefit. Because her symptoms improved so much she continued the practice, to the point where she joined a yoga teachers' course. This led her eventually to undertake a three-year meditation course. She now teaches both yoga and meditation professionally and has had many people enrolling in her classes as a result of chronic illness. Almost without fail, class members report benefits. She commented, when I interviewed her, that all her class members agree that you are either stressed out or at ease. At ease, the stress vanishes and you have less pain, and symptoms of illness are more manageable.

She went on to say that illness of any sort causes stress, which makes things worse and, of course, increases the stress. To ask anyone in this state to initiate a change of diet, do more exercise and do things differently can be daunting. When you practise yoga or meditation, you change in spite of yourself – your resistance is bypassed. The key is the practice of breathing. Breathing opens the door to change. On a physical level the relaxation induced by the breathing enables a message to get through to all the systems of the body to restore balance, so that such symptoms as headaches, generalized pain, back pain and other chronic conditions can improve. On an emotional and psychological level the relaxation induced by breathing and relaxed movement can open up people to talk, resolving long-standing issues, reducing isolation and easing feelings of depression.

I asked whether yoga is a good substitute for or an even better alternative to energetic exercise, especially for people with long-standing health problems. Rosanne replied,

> I believe so. Combining yoga breathing and movement changes the whole physiological process. Therapeutic movement is flowing, not forced as in intensive exercise. In yoga, as you move, the breath takes the strain and the body becomes ener-gized. Tension in the muscles is released so that blood flow improves, and of course the organs of the body work more effec-tively – restrictions to drainage and elimination are removed and hormones can be released to stimulate the body to work at its optimum level. It is a very healing process. You feel expanded and as a result problems do not overwhelm you.

We talked about the value of meditation, and Rosanne explained that we are made up of energy. Well-being is dependent on the energy of the heart – the heart has the strongest energy, even more powerful than that of the brain. This energy enables the body and mind to throw off stress and become relaxed and much more inclined to live in the moment.

Meditation can take you to a deeper level of intense awareness. You start by developing an awareness of the breathing process, and that awareness leads to increased awareness of everything in ourselves – body, thoughts, feelings – leading to an awareness of ourselves as part of a greater whole, the universe or cosmos. This is important for anyone who has become isolated and detached from other people because of illness or pain. If you have been stressed or under tension for a long time you may come to realize once more that you matter, you have your place in the world. With the release of tension many people have an emotional release and find themselves in tears with relief. It's like opening a gate when you've been locked in tension for so long. After all, pain, whether physical or emotional, is a lonely place. Meditation can help people accept their illness and be more realistic about the demands they put on themselves. They may accept that though they are no longer able to do the physical things they once did, they can still achieve on a different level.

Rosanne stressed that it is important to accept that healing may not be a once-and-for-all experience. We have many experiences – problems with work or relationships with children, siblings or elderly parents, financial difficulties, illness or even the death of other family members. All these can upset our equilibrium, cause stress, make our symptoms worse. In short, we experience personal and health setbacks. Our lifestyle may be incompatible with the illness: we may forget to pace ourselves, take on too much, lose control of our lives and try to live at the pace of those who have no health problems.

In following your plan for healing it is important to build on the breathing and relaxation exercises I have already described so that you can continue to restore the balance between your mind and body. As Rosanne indicated, maintaining this balance is not a once-and-for-all activity. It is a lifetime's work.

The following exercises are intended to start you off. As you become practised at them and, over a period of weeks, experience the benefits, you may find the confidence to use your imagination to develop them further to suit yourself.

Go into your breathing rhythm – in to a count of four, hold for a count of four and out for a count of six. If it helps, use the sound 'umm' as you breathe out until relaxation becomes established. As you become more relaxed, remember a very happy time in your life – something that made you feel good at the time. If you can, see that event in your mind's eye. Some people do find it difficult to visualize in this way but it does not matter. As you remember the event, remember how you felt, the things you heard, any smells associated with that memory. If you are able to see a picture, make it as big, clear and bright as possible. Note the clothes you or others are wearing and stay with the image and the memory for as long as possible.

While you are practising your breathing, try the following exercises.

1 Count your blessings; remember everything and everyone you feel grateful for.
2 Remember as many things as possible that have brought a smile to your face.

3 Smile and chuckle as you practise your relaxation breathing; this can be very energizing.
4 Remember those occasions that filled you with pride and made you really happy. Take note of your feelings. What sort of a day was it? Who was with you? Recall any sounds or smells associated with the memory. Often ladies I have worked with focus on the moment they held their baby for the first time.

Once you have started on this process you are beginning to use the skills involved in a very powerful healing technique: guided imagery or visualization, a tool often used by psychotherapists and hypnotherapists and in meditation. It is based on the idea that our imagination can help in the body's healing process. It is maintained that using visualization can bring about fundamental changes because when memories are evoked they become real and our bodies relive the original experience, reacting in the same way, producing the same hormones and chemicals into the bloodstream that lower the heart rate and blood pressure and reduce anxiety. This releases energy for healing. There are many records of people using their imagination to fight illness, and to reduce or even eliminate tumours. The idea is to imagine an army of good cells attacking the tumour and reducing it in size. At the beginning of the book I gave my own account of how I was encouraged in my healing by mentally changing black into white.

Freda's story

Some years ago, Freda came to see me. She explained that she had an inflammatory bowel condition. Her sister, a former colleague of mine, had recommended that she come to see me. Freda had a stressful job as a manager in a public organization. She was seen as the trouble-shooter and all problems landed on her desk. Her condition was very painful and at times embarrassing. She was not sleeping well and she felt that the medication she had been on for some years was not helpful. Her sister thought she should learn how to relax, hence her visit to me.

In exploring her history and lifestyle, it appeared that until her job had virtually taken over her life she had been keen on tapestry work, creating her own designs. She had a good eye for colour. I thought it might be a good idea to use this during her relaxation sessions so I asked her, when she was in a deeply relaxed state, to focus on the part of her that was unwell and to describe it. She described 'a horrible black and green mush'. I encouraged her to imagine changing this black and green mush into something more agreeable to her. She thought she would like to change it into a beautiful shade of pink, the colour she imagined a healthy bowel should be. In her collection of tapestry wools she had the precise shade so she imagined making up a drink in that shade. After three weeks practising deep relaxation every day and visualizing herself sipping the pink liquid, her symptoms were so much better, and she visualized her bowel fully restored to health. She was sleeping well and had so much more energy.

Other issues to consider

Eating for nutrition and healing

This section aims to present to you a number of issues that you may need to think about as you cope with your particular illness. I know from my experience working with people with chronic illness that many will not even consider changing eating and drinking habits of a lifetime unless their illness becomes life-threatening, like diabetes or heart disease. Even then, some decide not to make the effort, either because they do not believe that enjoyable food can be harmful, or because they would not dream of giving up their pleasures.

Following extensive research and clinical practice, there is no doubt that what we eat has a profound effect on our development through childhood and our ability to maintain health as we age. Rickets is a good example of a childhood nutritional deficiency. Old-time seamen suffered from scurvy on long sea voyages through lack of fruit and vegetables containing vitamin C. There is growing evidence that the foods we eat and the way they are prepared can have a direct effect in causing and exacerbating many current illnesses. Unless you have been on another planet you cannot have missed the media coverage and government pronouncements about obesity.

Type 2 diabetes, heart disease, bowel disorders and cancer, high blood pressure and breathing problems are commonly linked to the diet we 'enjoy' in the UK. Our national diet is increasingly dominated by processed and ready-to-eat meals and sauces, reconstituted meats, high concentrations of sugar and fat, fry-ups and a general lack of vegetables. There is no doubt that there is a need for everyone, wherever possible, to return to preparing meals within the home from fresh ingredients. Anyone with an illness will benefit by taking a fresh approach and having respect for his or her body. After all, our bodies have to last a long time but we risk shortening our lives because we have neglected or ill-treated them.

Car owners take pride in their vehicles and would not dream of feeding the car with the wrong fuel. Go to any motorway service station and you will see people with expensive and well-maintained cars going into the eating areas and choosing drinks high in sugar and carrying plates piled high with fried foods rich in animal fats. It is rare to see people choosing the vegetable or salad alternatives. I find it strange and unacceptable, when I visit my local leisure centre to carry out my health-promoting exercise, that as I leave I have to walk past a wall of vending machines selling crisps and fatty snack foods and sugary drinks of all kinds, including those in the guise of health drinks – worse still, a 10-foot-high poster for beer dominates the route to the car park. The centre is run by a local authority that sponsors the Health 4 Life scheme! (The Health 4 Life scheme aims to confront the problem of child obesity through work with schools and families; for further information, contact your local council offices.)

You may have determined that to help yourself cope with your chronic illness, you need to change what you eat and drink and the way you prepare your food. It can seem a daunting prospect but you do not have to change all at once. Research has shown that people who successfully make one simple change in any aspect of their lives can go on to build on that. Success breeds success. So, where do we begin if we know that our diet is endangering our health?

This section will help you work out for yourself the types and amounts of foods which will benefit your general health and your specific illness – but before we get to that, just think about making the one small change that will be the foundation of the healing that can be brought about by eating and drinking wisely. You can start by setting yourself a goal that you know at the outset you are capable of achieving. Perhaps I can help you by suggesting that you start each day with a glass of water, cold or warm, plain or garnished with a slice of lemon, whichever suits you. Alternatively, drink a cup of herbal tea, perhaps lemon and ginger. These are anti-inflammatory, refreshing and cleansing. Aim to do this for one week and in the meantime do not think about any other changes. At the end of the week, congratulate yourself for achieving your goal and take stock of how you feel. I know many people who say they feel better, more refreshed and cleansed as a result of this simple change.

Before going on to establish other goals, may I suggest you start a food diary, taking note of what and how much you eat and drink throughout each day, including alcohol. Do this for a week. It will help you to make your own assessment of your normal diet. To help you to make use of your food diary, at the end of the week study it and answer the following questions:

- Do you eat red meat, e.g. lamb, beef or pork, more than once a week?
- Do you eat sausages, bacon, black pudding or pies more than once a week?
- Do you eat cooked or tinned meats, e.g. ham, tongue, roast beef, pork, brawn, haslet or corned beef more than once a week?
- Do you eat processed tinned food without checking the list of ingredients?
- Do you eat ready-cooked meals from the freezer more than once a week?
- Do you eat deep-fried foods more than once a week?
- Do you send out for takeaways more than once a week?
- Do you have fried food most days of the week?
- Do you have more than two cups of tea or coffee a day?
- Do you have sugary and fizzy drinks more than twice a week?
- Do you eat cakes, pastries and crisps more than twice a week? Several at a time?
- Do you eat cheese more than once a week?
- Do you drink milk every day in addition to what you have in tea or coffee?
- Do you eat or drink any other dairy products (e.g. ice cream, yoghurt, cream, milk-based desserts, butter)?
- Do you add salt to your food at the table?
- Do you have sugary cereals, or add extra sugar to your breakfast cereals more than twice a week?
- Do you eat chocolates or sweets every day?

For every 'yes' answer, score 1 point. If you score 5 points or under, you are already seriously thinking about what you eat but you may wish to explore the size of your helpings and the number of meals you have in a day. If, however, you score 6 points or more it is time to take a serious look at your diet and consider making changes.

If your daily diet is heavily weighted in favour of the foods listed in the questionnaire then you owe it to yourself to put limits on the frequency you eat them and perhaps also limit the amount you eat.

Before going on to thinking about goals to set yourself, here are some more questions for you to think about:

- Do you have chronic illness?
- Are you taking prescription drugs?
- Are you also taking over-the-counter or recreational drugs?
- Are you overweight by more than 3 kg (7 lb)?
- Do you retain water, have swollen legs or ankles? Are you on prescription medication for these problems?
- Do you have any digestive problems, e.g. indigestion, heartburn, constipation, bloating, wind, acid reflux, hiatus hernia, irritable bowel syndrome?
- Do you take medication for any digestive problems?
- Do you have trouble sleeping?
- Do you often feel depressed or suffer from anxiety states?
- Do you take medication for sleep problems, anxiety or depression?
- Are you inactive for most of the day?
- Do you avoid the company of others?

If you have answered 'yes' to any of these questions, then it is even more important that you change your diet and your approach to food.

You may have found that since your activity level has been reduced as a result of your illness or pain you have put on a lot of weight. I know I did. Carrying extra weight is not helpful for anyone with a painful condition or with difficulties affecting joints so we owe it to ourselves to lighten the load.

When you were fully active you may have been able to eat whenever and whatever you fancied without this making any appreciable difference to your weight. When you are less mobile your food intake matters. If you do not move about much you do not burn off the calories and any surplus food goes to fat.

As we get older our metabolism slows down and we do not need so much food. Unfortunately the message has not got through to our appetite and we tend then to eat until that appetite is satisfied.

So now you are beginning to think of ways of making changes which directly improve your symptoms, and this is a good time to think about taking control of what you eat. You should by now see that you are able to control tension in your muscles and achieve relaxation. You may also have some ideas about making the best of your abilities and making use of resources around you.

The next step is to take control of your food – what you eat, when you eat, and how much you eat. I know this can be difficult if you do not do the shopping or the cooking, or if you live in a house where someone else has strong ideas about what is good for you. You may live in an institutional setting where you are fed a 'one size fits all' diet at regular and possibly frequent intervals. You must decide whether or not your diet suits you. Listen to your body – it will tell you. Everyone is different and our food needs are different. Perhaps this book will help you put your ideas across about what you should be eating. I am not saying it is easy, but it can be done and you will feel so much better on your new diet.

Make a start by limiting the amount of processed foods you eat and move on from there. By processed foods I mean cooked meats, pies and sausages, and this includes ready-wrapped meats and bacon from supermarkets. Ready-wrapped foods, in particular, contain sulphites and nitrites, chemicals that are used for preserving the colour and shelf-life but that are harmful to anyone who is allergic to aspirin or has an inflammatory illness. Tinned food is also highly processed and usually contains salt and sugar as preservatives and taste enhancers, but these are not in themselves nutritious and may be harmful to those with high blood pressure or diabetes. Ready-prepared meals, frozen or otherwise, are not to be recommended, especially for anyone coping with illness. Food used may be reconstituted and bulked out with starches and fats and also contain high quantities of sugar and salt. So, take care at all times and read the labels.

When I became ill, within a very short time I could not fasten my belt and felt very bloated. For some time I did nothing about it as I was more concerned about my pain. My family was concerned for my general health and worried about the rate at which I was expanding. As I began to become more skilful at controlling my pain, I had more energy and was able to focus more on the state of my body. The first step was to reduce the amount of food by changing from a large dinner plate to a much smaller plate and replacing my favourite mug with a dainty china teacup. Gradually I was able to move to having a substantial lunch, cutting out snacks and things like biscuits and crisps and just having a small meal such as egg on toast at about 6 p.m., then nothing more until the next morning. Without doing anything else I began slowly to lose weight.

As time went on and I got more interested in the question of nutrition. I took a serious look at what went into a meal. Fortunately as a family we all enjoyed home-cooked food and very rarely bought ready-cooked meals so it was not difficult to make changes. This is a big subject and a full account of these changes and the reasons for them are given in *The Chronic Pain Diet Book* (Sheldon Press, 2008), which was the result of 15 years of research.

As you become more motivated to change you will find it helpful to increase your fruit and vegetable intake (with the exception of potatoes). Try to reduce the intake of meat and animal fats. Steam or grill food rather than fry and if you find the taste is a bit bland experiment with herbs and spices rather than add extra salt. Eat 100 per cent wholemeal bread and cut out sugary cereals and drinks. Limit your alcohol intake: start off by drinking half pints rather than pints, singles rather than doubles and small glasses rather than large, but do not be tempted to increase the number of glasses to make up the volume.

Take stock of how much dairy produce you are eating (i.e. anything from the cow). There is a good deal of evidence from American studies that cow's milk should disappear from children's diet at about the age of five. It is claimed that continuing cow's milk beyond this age is at the root of many illnesses in adult life, including bowel problems, upper respiratory and chest problems, and even osteoporosis. It is even suggested that some cancers are related to the consumption of cow's milk. It is not recommended for people with arthritis or MS as there is evidence that people with these conditions have difficulty digesting and absorbing animal fats. There are many studies which indicate improvements after cow's milk is withdrawn from the diet.

Here is a quick quiz for you. Suppose you wished to limit your sugar intake, which of these foods would you choose as the best options?

- Bakery products
- Low-fat granola
- Sorbet
- Low-fat yoghurt
- Honey
- Brown rice syrup
- Corn syrup
- Dextrose
- Glucose
- Lactose
- Malt syrup
- Molasses
- Smoothies made from concentrates
- Ketchup
- Barbecue sauce
- Pasta sauce
- Reduced-fat salad dressing
- White bread
- White rice
- Potatoes
- Crisps
- Pasta
- Baked beans
- Energy bars
- Flavoured bottled water
- Sucrose

Beware all of them! They all contain sugar and starch in one form or another: for example, energy bars have a high sugar content and contain as many as 500 calories. Look out for bars with less than 200 calories. Most bakery products are rich in refined white flour and sugar. Granola may be low-fat but is full of sugar, as is low-fat yoghurt. They can have 30 g of sugar or other sweeteners. Be careful of so-called healthy yoghurts and drinks that claim to be fortified with Omega 3. They may have a small amount of Omega 3 but you still have to beware of the sugar content. Smoothies that are made from concentrates rather than whole fruit are rich in sugar, as is flavoured bottled water. Whatever you eat or drink, *never* take in more calories than you can burn off.

All the items listed contain empty calories that cause a surge in blood sugar but do not provide any nutrition. The surge in blood sugar lasts for no more than an hour or so and then you can be faced with a sudden drop in energy and perhaps feel the need to top up your blood sugar level once again by consuming more empty calories. Unless you are planning to do a 100-metre sprint or deliver a lorryload of coal immediately after consuming them, avoid these empty calories at all costs. If you do consume them when you have your favourite goodies, put strict limits on the amount you eat.

Try to choose foods that give you energy throughout the day, such as 100 per cent wholemeal bread, bananas, wholegrain rice or wholegrain pasta. If you are having sauces on your pasta, look for chopped tomatoes or passata and add your own herbs, fresh or dried. Get used to reading labels to see how much sugar is contained in tinned and packeted food. Sugar contributes to weight gain, increasing belly fat, fatty liver and obesity, which leads to diabetes or heart attack. Being overweight makes your body more resistant to the insulin your body produces naturally to break down the sugar, and this increases the risk of diabetes.

Excess sugar in the blood also creates more acid in the system and this contributes to inflammation throughout the body. Anyone with an inflammatory disease will experience more setbacks as a result. People with strong cravings for sugar, or having difficulty in regulating the amount of sugar in their diet, may benefit from a course of chromium tablets. Of course, if you suspect you have diabetes, or have been diagnosed, then these tablets are not recommended and you should always seek the advice of your doctor.

In recent years a considerable body of evidence has shown that there is a link between meat-eating, cancer and heart disease. The human body is unable to deal with excessive amounts of animal fats and cholesterol. Anyone who has a meat-centred diet is likely to accumulate excess cholesterol, which clogs up the inner walls of the arteries and constricts the flow of blood to the heart and can lead to high blood pressure, heart disease and stroke. Research suggests a link between excessive meat-eating and cancer of the colon, rectum, breast and uterus. It is also suggested that the consumption of animal fats can contribute to and exacerbate such illnesses as arthritis; as in heart disease, the build-up of cholesterol in the arteries restricts the blood flow to the joints and contributes to inflammation. Think of it as being like grease that, when poured down the sink, sticks to the pipes; over time the grease becomes so thick that it makes the pipes very narrow and you get a blockage.

In the case of MS, many people have difficulty absorbing animal fats. People with arthritis and other inflammatory diseases also have problems with food absorption. In addition, many food allergies and intolerances are said to arise from the inability of the digestive system to process certain foods. As we get older our bodies produce fewer of the enzymes necessary for the complete digestion of food. As this happens, absorption problems can get worse. Many nutrition therapists recommend that the system can be improved by taking a course of digestive enzymes to help cope with the processing of fats and carbohydrates. Because the digestive process continues into the bowel it is possible that still more help is needed to avoid inflammation and possible cancer risks so it is recommended that uncooked green vegetable matter is eaten every day. For this reason I grow cut-and-come-again salads in my garden.

Food has a direct bearing on inflammation and therefore on pain levels. I am unable to take painkillers and anti-inflammatories based on aspirin and therefore must use food to help me control inflammation and pain. Inflammation increases if, in addition to excessive sugar, the diet includes animal fats such as those found in red meat, dairy products and saturated cooking oils. The safest of cooking oils is olive oil but sunflower oil can be used if you prefer a lighter oil. Olive oil described as 'light' is no different from any other olive oil, except in colour.

Many people who have chronic pain or arthritis are also food sensitive. Their sensitivity may have a direct effect on their pain and on their illness. It can also produce inflammation and swelling in the digestive tract which limits the ability of the digestive system to digest food completely. If you are unaware that you have a sensitivity to a particular food, then continued use of that food will further compromise the digestive tract, causing even more inflammation around the joints and, of course, exacerbating pain and mobility problems.

Stress resulting from coping with pain or illness may be a constant in your life. It may increase as a result of lack of sleep and fatigue. When you are under constant stress, cortisol, the stress hormone, is secreted into the bloodstream leading directly to an increase in your appetite. You may also seek out comfort foods as you try to cope with your stress – and they are not usually the most healthy. There is evidence that 25 per cent of people taking anti-depressants over a long period gain weight. The weight gain could also result from the depression itself. It can be difficult to restore a balance in your body because both the depression and the medication can influence your appetite and how much you eat. As your depression eases you may also find that your appetite increases and the amount and types of food you choose to eat have changed, adding to your weight problem. If this is happening to you then you must seek the help of your doctor.

Anti-inflammatory steroid medications known as corticosteroids, often prescribed for conditions such as asthma, lupus and arthritis, have the unfortunate side effect of causing weight gain as a result of fluid retention and increased appetite. If the medicine is continued in increasing doses over a long period, the weight gain is exacerbated.

Your illness may mean that you are prescribed mood-altering drugs or you may be on medication for migraine, high blood pressure or diabetes. Unfortunately these may also have an effect on your weight. If you have tried to stop smoking you have probably gained weight as a result of increasing your calorie intake. As a hypnotherapist, I would have considered myself to have failed professionally if any of my clients had put on weight as a result of giving up smoking. Putting on weight should not be a direct result of giving up smoking. Smoking is a habit and so is comfort eating. Remove one habit and many people replace it with the other. Often, under hypnosis, I suggested deep, diaphragmatic breathing followed by a glass of water as a good substitute for cigarettes. It worked more often than not.

There are, of course, medical conditions such as an under-active thyroid which can cause weight gain. If you do feel you have a weight problem, you may want to discuss it with your medical advisers or dietitian.

Alcohol is high in calories and can also lead to weight gain. Another factor about alcohol that you need to take into account is that although it may appear to relieve your pain and lift your mood temporarily, there is always a 'kick-back' effect and your pain levels can increase rapidly. I have known a number of people with pain problems who have tried alcohol therapy only to find its long-term effects do a great deal of damage to their health.

Good food equals good medicine

My solution to the problem of reducing pain and inflammation without drugs, in addition to exercise and relaxation, is a diet rich in vegetables and oily fish such as salmon, herring, sardines and mackerel. These help the body produce a number of anti-inflammatory compounds. I also have my own special remedy: arrowroot.

Arrowroot

Arrowroot is available from the home-baking department of any good supermarket. It has been used since Roman times, generally as a food for invalids and babies and to cope with the symptoms of stomach and bowel problems. It is soothing to the whole of the digestive system. It is my first line of defence against inflammation and I take it knowing that it reduces internal swelling and eliminates excessive water. You may have found for yourself that water retention increases the inflammation in your body.

Because it is not a drug, arrowroot causes none of the nasty side effects that often accompany drugs. Arrowroot itself is tasteless. You may know it as a thickener for soups, stews or fruit dishes or used by itself or with cornflour to make a dessert flavoured with vanilla or chocolate. I make it into a drink, using a heaped teaspoonful mixed to a paste with half an inch of cold water, then adding hot water up to a cupful, stirring gently until it turns clear.

The following foods are not only nutritious but make good medicine if included in home-cooked food on a daily basis.

Almonds and avocado

These are known to be effective in helping to reduce high blood pressure. Include a daily intake of four or five almonds in your daily diet. You need to eat them every day for them to be most effective. However, watch your teeth! If this worries you, try toasted flaked or ground almonds instead. Ground almonds can also be used as a healthy substitute for the less healthy processed flours in baking recipes and soups. They are ideal for people on a wheat-free or gluten-free diet.

Avocado can be added to salads or even used as a vegetable. A more unusual use is in the following recipe for Avocado Chocolate Mousse. I am including this because I found it to be a truly healing experience to have this treat, having been unable to tolerate dairy products for many years. It is food for my mind, body and spirit!

Avocado Chocolate Mousse with Strawberries

Serves 2

1½ ripe medium-sized avocados (in our house we use two because we never know what to do with half an avocado, and besides it gives us a bigger helping!)
25 g good-quality cocoa powder
25 ml water
50 ml Sweet Freedom*
2 handfuls strawberries thinly sliced, for decoration

Place all ingredients except strawberries into a blender and blend until smooth, scraping the sides down a few times while blending. Spoon the mousse into two small bowls and top with the strawberries. (I leave off the strawberries because of my allergy to them – but it tastes just as good.)

* Sweet Freedom is a 100 per cent fruit syrup sold as a sweetener with a low glycaemic index so it is ideal for people with diabetes, those who wish to lose weight and people who have an intolerance to most sugars. It is sold in Morrison's and Waitrose supermarkets.

Avocados can also be made into guacamole which is a healthy addition to your diet.

Guacamole

2 avocados
1 teaspoon grated onion
1 teaspoon lemon juice
2 teaspoons extra virgin olive oil
A pinch of cayenne pepper or chilli powder
Seasoning as required

Peel and mash the avocados well. Blend in all the other ingredients and beat thoroughly.

Onions, shallots, spring onions and chives

These are valuable to anyone with arthritis, rheumatic pain or period pain. They ease fluid retention and promote the elimination of urea, a chemical produced by the body as part of waste elimination. A build-up of urea can make inflammatory conditions worse.

Olive oil

This has nutritional and medicinal qualities. It contains vitamins A and E and the minerals phosphorus, potassium and manganese as well as anti-oxidants. The oil is useful in balancing cholesterol levels in the blood and preventing fatty deposits being laid down in the arteries, and as a consequence reduces heart disease, blood clots and strokes. Anyone with chronic pain and arthritic conditions needs to have a good blood flow to all parts of the body and this is where olive oil plays its part.

If you are changing your diet to reduce the amount of saturated fats you use in cooking or consume in ready-made foods, then olive oil is a good substitute. When using it for frying, use a little olive oil and the same amount of water. Olive oil is helpful in easing the ravages of stress and poor food absorption in the digestive system. It is often recommended as a remedy for constipation which results from the use of prescription medicines. A dessertspoonful of cold-pressed extra virgin olive oil can be taken either by itself or drizzled on a piece of bread.

Ginger

Ginger has well-known anti-inflammatory effects. It helps block the chemicals that trigger inflammation. Studies indicate that people with migraine can be helped by taking half to one teaspoonful of ground ginger each day. I take it in this way from time to time and find that it helps in my battle against inflammation, contributing to the reduction of swelling and joint stiffness.

Since digestive problems seem to accompany many of the common pain disorders, it is worth using ginger as a digestive aid. It works just as well in the powdered form as with the fresh root form. Besides reducing inflammation in the gut it reduces nausea and has a calming effect on the stomach and bowel, thus promoting healing.

I also use root ginger liberally in cooking, sliced very thinly or grated. It is particularly good in Chinese dishes or added to marmalades or jams. My first cup of tea in the morning is lemon and ginger.

It is worth trying it for yourself over a period of three months before making a judgement. Any remedy such as this needs time. It is not an instant fix – it is the cumulative effect that is important. There is no fear of overdosing or side effects.

Turmeric

The effects of turmeric are similar to those of ginger in that it has a calming effect on the digestive system and the bowel and is cooling and anti-inflammatory. There are research indications that turmeric may be effective in preventing some forms of cancer.

Broccoli

Broccoli has a high vitamin C and mineral content so it contributes to the nutritional value of any meal. Fortunately, it is my favourite vegetable. As a bonus I find it helpful in combating fluid retention and inflammation, and consequently it is one of the weapons I use in reducing my pain.

100 per cent wholemeal flour

Other flours may contain large quantities of refined white flour and some brown flours are merely refined white flour with added colour, so look out for 100 per cent wholemeal bread if you are not baking your own. Fibre is an essential part of a healthy diet and 100 per cent wholemeal flour, along with vegetables, is an ideal source.

Wholegrain rice

Wholegrain rice is another good source of fibre. It is free from gluten and lactose as well as providing the body with slow-release carbohydrates to ensure a long-lasting energy supply. Refined, polished white rice has little to commend it as a food. It is a filler, low in fibre, and is a poor provider of long-lasting energy. All the goodness has been removed in the processing.

Keep moving

Years ago I suddenly realized that the most important way for me to cope with my illness and my pain was to adopt the motto 'Keep moving'. For me, 'Keep moving' means keeping out of bed when pain strikes, not sitting too long, and doing exercise that does not exhaust me but keeps my joints supple and flexible and keeps my heart in a healthy condition. Just because we have illness in one part of our body does not mean that we have to neglect the rest of it. In fact, it means that we have to strengthen our weaker parts and ensure the most healthy parts of ourselves remain healthy and strong, because they will be taking on an added burden. There are probably only a handful of illnesses where exercise and activity is expressly forbidden, so before you embark on any form of exercise find out from your doctor whether your illness is part of that handful.

Keeping moving does not always mean formal exercise but it does mean that throughout the day you monitor yourself, making sure that you do not lie in bed too long, no matter how you feel, that you do not sit too long and that you climb stairs or steps whenever possible. If you have a garden, work in it. Do as much housework as you can, while at the same time ensuring that you do not get exhausted. Aim for a balance between healthy physical activity, rest and relaxation. Take every opportunity to stretch and move your arms and legs. People with chronic pain can easily develop a fear of movement; I have been there myself, and have only been able to get out of that situation with the help of professionals who have ensured I have followed a programme of progressive gentle exercise that has focused on working every part of my body. Such a programme is outlined in my books *Coping Successfully with Pain* and *The Chronic Pain Handbook*.

If you find yourself in a position where you fear to do anything at all because of your illness, then you really must talk to your doctor and ask about a pain management course. Otherwise, enquire whether there is a suitable physiotherapy course in your area which tackles rehabilitation for people who have had strokes, or who have arthritis, MS, lupus, fibromyalgia, osteoporosis or balance problems. The main thing is that you make sure the programme is suitable for you in your present physical condition, and that a full assessment of this will be made before you start. Many of these programmes take place, not in hospital, but in local leisure centres.

What sort of exercise should you be doing? How long is a piece of string?

Take the example of Jim, who struggled to find a balance between his need to carry on being 'one of the boys', playing sport and drinking, and his diabetes. What and how much to do is something you are going to have to work out for yourself, but if you are in any doubt at all get some advice from a medical or sports medicine practitioner. Bodies were made to move and they feel better as a result of the activity. See how much better you feel if you get out of your chair and move around to the rhythm of the music on the radio. Just move, sway, swing and let your arms move freely. If you get out of breath, so much the better. Aim to move in a way that leaves you able to talk quite comfortably as you do so. Even better, sing or hum along to the music as you move. Make it a fun activity. There is no reason why your exercise should be looked on as one stage removed from torture!

Whatever you choose to do, start slowly and remember age is no barrier. It should feel good, increase your energy and build self-confidence. If you choose walking or cycling it is helpful to team up with a partner and make the exercise part of a pleasurable trip or day out. I often struggle to find ways of exercising on cold, wet days in winter (or even in a British summer!) so I have an exercise bike at home as a back-up.

There is nothing like a good stre-e-e-etch!

Many of us have a limited range of motion because of muscle or nerve problems, or because we have been inactive for a long time. Stretching is an ideal way to get moving again, paying attention to our breathing as we move and taking care to stretch every part of our body. You may need the help of others to get you started but it is easy to get hold of a suitable programme from books or DVDs or perhaps even from your practice nurse. Stretching with assistance is often used for people recovering from strokes. There is a growing practice for elderly people and those recovering from illness to be referred to a group to do chair exercises.

However, a note of caution: even these simple, undemanding exercises may not be suitable for everyone. There needs to be a thorough assessment of everyone's capabilities and physical condition before starting, especially if people have nerve and muscle problems.

Make use of community resources

If you have a swimming pool nearby, make use of it, and if there are any special hydrotherapy classes these are well worth joining, especially if you have arthritis, MS or hip, knee or joint problems.

We are fortunate that most of us live within easy reach of a gym or leisure centre. If you are worried about wearing shorts in public, there is no problem. Exercise as I do, in tracksuit trousers. If there is no special physiotherapist-supervised exercise programme, it is safe to put your trust in the hands of the centre supervisors who will devise a programme suitable for you and your condition. They will make sure that you start slowly and they will explain how to use the machines. Often older people or those with medical conditions or in receipt of benefits can get a discount or even attend free of charge.

If you wish to combine exercise with social activity look out for the various kinds of dance and movement clubs or classes in your area. You might just want to attend and watch for a time to see if it suits you. I am thinking of such things as line dancing, zumba, aerobics, Pilates, t'ai chi, yoga and, as it used to be in my youth, old-time and country dancing! All of these things will make you feel better, happier and much more alive.

Yoga

Rosanne and Sarah, in their interviews, told us of the benefits they had gained from the practice of yoga which has specific advantages for those with a chronic condition. It is in fact suitable for everyone, old and young, healthy or sick. It has been practised for 4,000 years, and during that time millions of people have either maintained their health or regained their emotional, spiritual and physical well-being through it. The focus is on developing awareness of the body and our breathing. In yoga, movement is coordinated with breathing as a range of postures are carried out. In many ways it is a form of meditation, as to do it properly one has to become skilled in the practice of awareness.

Do not be put off by some of the extreme postures that may be demonstrated by expert practitioners. Everyone starts off with very simple, uncomplicated, calm movements. Many of the postures are done in a lying or sitting position, so people with certain medical conditions need not be excluded. It is also possible to use supports such as a chair or a wall. As Rosanne explained, we do not always have to do some form of intensive, aerobic exercise to get healthy benefits. What is important is the breathing, coordinated with movement, carried out without strain on a regular daily basis. In this way it becomes part of your life and it will not take long before you are able to appreciate the benefits to your health and your ability to move more freely.

T'ai chi

T'ai chi is really a martial art, a form of training intended to increase the flow of life energy (chi) throughout the body. Like yoga, the movements are synchronized with breathing. Rather than adopting postures, the discipline encourages graceful, flowing movements. It is often described as a form of moving meditation. It has become very popular throughout the world as a form of exercise for older people. It involves no strain whatsoever and is particularly helpful for people to overcome balance problems and for those with limited ability to stand for long periods. It has been found to be helpful for those with heart problems.

Support from alternative and complementary therapies

Never feel that you are abandoned. From time to time you may need help from your doctor or the National Health Service in the form of adjustment of medication or perhaps physiotherapy but *always consult your doctor if your symptoms change.*

Listen to your body

It can be very expensive seeking help outside the NHS, especially if you entertain the hope of a complete cure. This is why we must constantly boost our inner resources, keep as fit and healthy as possible and aim for the best quality of life that we can.

From time to time you may need help that is not available on the NHS. For the most part complementary or alternative practitioners are well trained and highly skilled. You will have plenty of time to talk and you will not feel rushed. The following information describes the kind of help available and I am sure your medical adviser will be only too pleased to discuss any of these with you. Just let me say that it is not unusual nowadays for doctors to recommend a complementary therapist to their patients. On occasions I have benefited from help from various medical and complementary practitioners, and before I retired as a psychotherapist and hypnotherapist I was able in my turn to help many people with pain, depression, anxiety and other chronic illnesses.

Electrical stimulation

Strictly speaking this form of treatment will be prescribed by a consultant or GP. I have included the topic here because apart from an initial trial you will probably have to purchase the equipment if it suits you.

Transcutaneous Nerve Stimulation (TENS) involves stimulating tissue with electrical current. The device used is small, about the size of a mobile phone, and is usually referred to as a TENS machine. You have no need to be frightened about the idea of electrical current: the amount transmitted is painless and mild. The current is conveyed along thin wires through patches placed on the skin to stimulate specific nerves, and generates heat which helps relieve muscle pain and promote circulation. It is also believed to stimulate the production of natural painkillers.

The device has been widely used for many years for the relief of pain. It is somewhat of an advance on the electric eels the Romans used for the same purpose. As far back as the period between the two world wars, a patent hand-cranked electrical stimulation machine, which required you to hold two brass electrodes in your hands while someone else turned the handle, was widely advertised for the relief of headaches.

TENS is found to be very helpful in childbirth and people with chronic pain have also benefited from its use. It is still recommended to people who attend pain clinics. However, it is not suitable for everyone and generally the pain clinic will lend you a machine for about six weeks to see how you get on with it. Unlike drug treatment there are no dangerous and uncomfortable side effects, the treatment of which can be extremely costly. Until recently, TENS machines were rather expensive but now they can be bought on the internet and in some of the high street chemists for under £20.

I used one every day for about 17 years and was grateful for the pain relief it gave as I am allergic to all painkillers based on aspirin. Fortunately the continuous use of pain management techniques means that I need to use a TENS only occasionally, when I am subjecting myself to additional demands such as going on long journeys when I might have to sit or stand for long periods.

The TENS machine is not recommended to be used when driving. Neither is it recommended for people who have pacemakers fitted.

Acupuncture

This is an ancient Chinese system of medicine that involves inserting fine needles at specific points on the body. It is generally safe, with few adverse effects. A number of pain clinics in the UK use acupuncture, and in recent years it has become almost a mainstream treatment, used in many hospitals. Research has revealed that acupuncture produces benefits in a number of medical conditions, including pain. It has an effect on the brain and nerves and can stimulate the production of endorphins, the body's natural pain-relieving chemicals.

Acupressure is an alternative form of treatment which does not involve the use of needles but instead uses finger pressure on the points where needles are usually inserted.

Chiropractic

Chiropractic manipulation, developed about 150 years ago, focuses on musculoskeletal disorders and research indicates that it is very effective in cases of low back pain. The idea of chiropractic treatment is that the body has a natural ability to keep itself healthy and this is helped if normal nerve function can be restored. Misaligned vertebrae interfere with nerve function so treatment involves using the hands to move vertebrae into their proper positions. Apart from those with low back pain, people with recurring headaches and fibromyalgia may also be helped.

I have a chiropractic check-up once or twice a year, particularly following times when I have stumbled or tripped. Stumbling is one of the consequences of spinal stenosis, and the jarring can exacerbate the problems caused by narrow nerve canals which are characteristic of the condition. The treatment effectively eases the pressure on the nerves.

Massage

A wide variety of styles and techniques exist to manipulate muscles, ligaments and other soft tissue. The aim of massage is to relieve muscle tightness and spasms, increase blood flow, stimulate or relax the nervous system, and stimulate the release of toxic substances from the body in order to reduce stress. It is used frequently for pain relief. It can be practised by a qualified massage therapist or a physiotherapist. I can vouch for its effectiveness, especially in reaching areas deep in the body where tightness needs to be relieved.

Gentle massage techniques are easy to learn and research has shown self-massage can relieve pain and produce a feeling of well-being. It is a mutually healing activity when practised between couples who wish to maintain a sense of intimacy during illness.

Biofeedback

Biofeedback machines are used in clinical settings to help in the diagnosis and treatment of a number of medical conditions, such as chronic pain or high blood pressure, without the use of drugs. Biofeedback involves the use of electronic instruments that measure a number of physiological functions such as pulse rate, muscle tension and brainwave activity.

It also measures the galvanic skin response: that is, how much the sweat on the surface of your skin changes its resistance to electrical impulses. When people are tense, stressed, excited or thinking worrying thoughts, the amount of sweat produced is altered. Measurements are taken by the use of sensors, usually attached to the fingertips.

The machine gives out either a visual display or a sound signal as changes take place. With guidance, patients pay attention to the signals and gradually learn to alter their responses, usually by changing their breathing pattern or controlling their thoughts.

Versions of the biofeedback machine have been designed for home use for educational, entertainment and leisure purposes. I use one which links into my computer and takes me step by step through deep breathing exercises and guided meditations. It is a very useful aid for my own relaxation and pain control, but I also find it very entertaining because my progress is indicated as I successfully complete a series of challenges, similar to video games. The only way to win is to breathe properly and relax completely. In this way I am trained to change my physiological responses, and consequently my pain, without effort.

When I was working with patients I often used a simple biofeedback machine to help those who were unsure of hypnotherapy to understand how they could be in control of their responses without the intervention of a therapist. There is a lot of evidence that biofeedback is a relaxation technique that is scientifically proven to have a powerful, positive effect on your emotional and physical well-being as well as being an effective form of treatment for pain.

Just a note of caution – if you are using a machine for the first time without guidance it is easy to become impatient and try too hard, especially if the machine emits audio signals. When this happens, relaxation does not follow. The whole essence of the machine is that you learn to adopt a slow, deep breathing rhythm, so do not be discouraged.

There is a wide range of biofeedback machines available to the public and the internet is a good place to start your search. Some machines can be quite expensive but the cost compares favourably with the cost of, say, a private visit to the dentist.

Hypnotherapy

For the last 50 or 60 years hypnotherapy has been accepted by the medical profession as a legitimate therapeutic procedure. It is used in many hospitals and in dentistry. The practice of hypnosis has in the past been associated with stage entertainment, usually showing people making fools of themselves under what is claimed to be 'a hypnotic state'. Therapeutic hypnosis stresses that at all times people in the hypnotic state remain under their own control. During therapy, a hypnotized person enters into a state of altered consciousness, guided by the therapist. A similar state is achieved if a person is practising visualization, meditation or even day-dreaming. Under the hypnotic state a person is less likely to resist suggestions for change and more likely to take on board helpful ideas for improvement.

Hypnotherapy has been found useful in treating undesirable behaviour or habits, such as phobias, smoking or food or sugar addiction, in managing anger and emotional and psychological problems, in alleviating symptoms of various medical conditions such as eczema and in the relief of chronic pain. When working with chronic pain patients I always found it worthwhile to teach them self-hypnosis, which is a very successful way to treat chronic pain. The relaxation activities in this book will have given you some experience of learning and applying the skill of self-hypnosis.

Reflexology

First practised by the ancient Egyptians and Chinese, the therapeutic foot or hand massage known as reflexology is a popular non-invasive complementary therapy. It is based on the principle that the reflexes found in areas of the hands and feet correspond to all the organs, systems and glands in the body. If you look at any book on reflexology you will see an illustration showing the feet as a mini map of the whole body. While effective in treating a wide range of conditions, reflexology does not set out to heal specific illnesses. The aim of reflexology treatment is to produce a state of relaxation and to restore balance between all the different systems of the body.

The therapist uses fingers and thumbs to apply gentle pressure. Through this pressure it is possible to detect tiny deposits and imbalances. Working on these points enables the therapist to release blockages, restore the flow of energy and assist in the restoration of balance between the various body systems. As a result, tension and stress can be eased, sleep patterns improved and pain levels reduced.

From my own experience and that of others I know it can induce deep relaxation. Anyone undergoing the treatment should not make any plans for the rest of the day. I fall into a deep sleep for several hours following each treatment and wake up thoroughly refreshed and pain-free for weeks at a time. I cannot guarantee that this will happen every time and to every person, of course. We will all react in our own ways to the treatment and it may not be suitable for everyone, but it is worth a try!

Spiritual healing

This is not to be confused with spiritualism or the dramatic exhibitions of 'healing' that you may see on television 'God spots'. The person is not asked to have any religious faith. Practitioners do not advertise nor do they charge for their services, but they will accept donations. Spiritual healers believe that all healing comes from within and that they act as a 'channel' to enable a person to heal him or herself. They are most effective in removing emotional blockages to healing, removing anxiety in the person and his or her loved ones. This results in a surge of energy and feelings of well-being which help you to take charge of your life again.

Healers are often said to have 'healing hands' which generate a lot of heat in the parts of the body of the person being treated. The hands are also used to scan the body for imbalances. The healer might detect energy blockages and leave his or her hands on the body for a while to promote release. In working closely with the patient the healer might become aware of emotional blockages which need to be released.

There are many techniques that might be used, including powerful visualizations. A healer was part of the therapeutic team at the Walton Hospital pain management course in Liverpool and was acknowledged by all to be a real help in the treatment of chronic pain. I've described my own experience of healing at the start of this book, although again I cannot guarantee that everyone would have a similar response.

Osteopathy

Osteopathy was developed in the United States in the middle of the nineteenth century. The discipline is based on the idea that the musculoskeletal system is central to the health and well-being of the body. By correcting problems in the body's structure using manipulation, its ability to function and to heal itself can be greatly improved.

Misalignment in the body's structure may result from muscle injuries, tension and poor posture and may also impair health by blocking the free flow of blood and lymphatic fluids. The osteopathic manipulation is designed to increase mobility and release muscle tension. Research indicates that people with low back pain and arthritis need fewer pain relievers and anti-inflammatory drugs than those people who are treated conventionally.

Having read the above descriptions you will have no doubt gathered that 'all roads lead to Rome', inasmuch as successful treatment produces deep relaxation and a calm mind – the very essence of this handbook.

This survey of complementary treatments does not cover everything on offer but these are the ones most commonly available in most areas of the country. Many people choose a therapist through word of mouth but you would be wise to consult the Institute for Complementary and Natural Medicine (see Useful addresses). The Institute keeps a register of all qualified complementary practitioners.

If you choose a complementary practitioner then make sure you do not agree to have treatment on an open-ended basis. At the outset make it clear that you would like to try no more then three treatment sessions. Three sessions should give a clear indication whether or not you are getting any benefit. The words 'I would like to see you again next week . . . next month . . .' should be a warning for you to be asking how many treatments the practitioner anticipates before you feel any benefit. (The same applies to *all* medical consultants.) Open-ended commitments can cost you a lot of money and may not necessarily be helpful to you.

A final thought

This book has been illustrated with stories of my attempts to come to terms with my illness, to find ways of coping, to achieve peace of mind and to live a life I can be proud of. Other people's stories have been used to show how they have been healed so that they too could live a full and satisfying life.

Why not tell your own story of your attempt to find healing? You will find it will make a contribution to your own well-being. It will show where you started your journey and highlight the pitfalls and triumphs. You may not have ambitions to publish your story, but writing it and sharing it with those close to you and others in your situation will make sure your experience and learning are not wasted.

Useful addresses

Allergy UK
Planwell House
LEFA Business Park
Edgington Way
Sidcup
Kent DA14 5BH
Tel.: 01322 619898 (helpline)
Website: www.allergyuk.org

Arthritis Care
18 Stephenson Way
London NW1 2HD
Tel.: 020 7380 6500 (general information); 0808 800 4050 (helpline, 10 a.m. to 4 p.m., Monday to Friday)
Website: www.arthritiscare.org.uk
This charity provides community-based management courses in addition to its other resources.

Backcare
16 Elmtree Road
Teddington
Middlesex TW11 8ST
Tel.: 020 8977 5474 (9 a.m. to 4 p.m., Monday to Thursday)
Helpline: 0845 130 2704
Website: www.backcare.org.uk

Institute for Complementary and Natural Medicine
Can-Mezzanine
32–36 Loman Street
London SE1 0EH
Tel.: 020 7922 7980
Website: www.icnm.org.uk
Provides information on all professionally qualified and registered complementary practitioners.

Institute for Optimum Nutrition
Avalon House
72 Lower Mortlake Road
Richmond
Surrey TW9 2JY
Tel.: 020 8614 7800
Website: www.ion.ac.uk
An educational charity which seeks to advance nutritional education and awareness to the general public and to health professionals. Publishes *Optimum Nutrition* magazine.

Pain Association Scotland
Suite D, Moncrieffe Business Centre
Friarton Road
Perth PH2 8DF
Tel.: 01738 629503 (admin)
Freephone: 0800 783 6059 (general enquiries, 8 a.m. to 4.30 p.m., Monday to Friday)
Website: www.painassociation.com
This charity provides a service throughout Scotland for people with pain. A relaxation/guided imagery course devised and delivered by Neville Shone is available on 3 CDs at a nominal charge, only from Pain Association Scotland. All proceeds from sales of these CDs go to the charity's work.

Pain Concern UK
Unit 1–3
62–66 Newcraighall Road
Fort Kinnaird
Edinburgh EH15 3HS
Tel.: 0131 669 5951 (office, 10 a.m. to 4 p.m., Monday to Friday)
Helpline: 0300 123 0789 (freephone)
Website: www.painconcern.org.uk
This group is run by people who are themselves coping with chronic pain.

I strongly suggest that if you have access to a computer you visit YouTube and search for Exercises for pain; Exercises for back pain; Stretching exercises; or Yoga exercises. Each of these searches will produce exercise demonstrations that I have found to be very useful, and that I myself have been able to perform without difficulty.

Biofeedback machines: An internet search will provide many websites where these are on sale; I obtained my own via <www.wilddivine.com>.

Further reading and resources

Books

Barnard, Neal, *Foods that Fight Pain: Revolutionary new strategies for maximum pain relief*, London: Bantam, 1999.

Buckley, Tessa, *The Multiple Sclerosis Diet Book: Help and advice for this chronic condition*, London: Sheldon Press, 2007.

Campbell, Don, *The Mozart Effect: Tapping the power of music to heal the body, strengthen the mind and unlock the creative spirit*, London: Hodder & Stoughton, 2001.

Center for Integrative Medicine at Duke University, *The Encyclopedia of New Medicine: Conventional and alternative medicine for all ages*, Emmaus, Pennsylvania: Rodale Books International, 2006.

Cerney, J. V., *Acupuncture without Needles: Do-it-yourself acupressure, the simple, at-home treatment for lasting relief from pain*, Upper Saddle River, New Jersey: Prentice Hall, 1974 and 1999.

Craggs-Hinton, Christine, *The Fibromyalgia Healing Diet*, London: Sheldon Press, 2008.

Greener, Mark and Craggs-Hinton, Christine, *The Diabetes Healing Diet*, London: Sheldon Press, 2012.

Holford, Patrick, *The Optimum Nutrition Bible*, London: Piatkus, 1998.

Melzack, R. and Wall, P. D., *The Puzzle of Pain*, London: Penguin Books, 1997.

Nown, Graham and Wells, Chris, *The Pain Relief Handbook: Self-help methods for managing pain*, London: Vermilion, 1996.

Rossman, M., *Guided Imagery for Self-Healing: An essential resource for anyone seeking wellness*, San Francisco, New World Library, 2000.

Shone, Neville, *Coping Successfully with Pain*, London: Sheldon Press, 2002.

Shone, Neville, *The Chronic Pain Diet Book*, London: Sheldon Press, 2008.

Shone, Neville, *The Pain Management Handbook: Your personal guide*, London: Sheldon Press, 2011.

Spero, David, *The Art of Getting Well: A five-step plan for maximising health when you have a chronic illness*, Alameda, California: Hunter House, 2002.

Weil, Dr Andrew, *Eating Well for Optimum Health*, New York: TimeWarner, 2001.

Whitfield, Charles, *Healing the Child Within: Discovery and recovery for adult children of dysfunctional families*, Deerfield Beach, Florida: Health Communications, 1991.

Websites

livingwithcfs.workpress.com (a good link for those with chronic fatigue syndrome)
www.actionforme.org.uk
www.arthritiscare.org.uk
www.bhf.org.uk

www.chronicpaininfo.org
www.diabetes.org.uk
www.headway.org.uk
www.health.com (see articles on diet and rheumatoid arthritis pain)
www.lupus.org.uk
www.meassociation.org.uk (for ME and CFS patients)
www.meresearch.org.uk
www.mssociety.org.uk
www.self-help.org.uk (provides links to many self-help groups and charities, including obesity support)
www.stroke.org.uk
www.ukfibromyalgia.com (see article on 'Diet and lifestyle' within 'Nutrition' section)
www.who.int/topics/chronic_diseases/en/

Index